Rheumatology

a case-based approach to management

Rheumatology

a case-based approach to management

Nidhi Sofat
BSc, MBBS, PhD, PGCert, FHEA, FRCP
Professor of Rheumatology, St George's,
University of London
St George's University Hospitals NHS Trust

Zoe Rutter-Locher
BSc, MBBS, MRCP, PGCert, MSc
Rheumatology Trainee Registrar
Guy's and St Thomas' NHS Trust

Helen Oakley
BSc, MCSP
Advanced Physiotherapy Practitioner
Physiotherapy Department, St George's University Hospitals NHS Trust

Scion

© **Scion Publishing Ltd, 2021**

ISBN 9781911510642

First published 2021

A CIP catalogue record for this book is available from the British Library.

Scion Publishing Limited

The Old Hayloft, Vantage Business Park, Bloxham Road, Banbury OX16 9UX, UK
www.scionpublishing.com

Important Note from the Publisher

The information contained within this book was obtained by Scion Publishing Ltd from sources believed by us to be reliable. However, while every effort has been made to ensure its accuracy, no responsibility for loss or injury whatsoever occasioned to any person acting or refraining from action as a result of information contained herein can be accepted by the authors or publishers.

Readers are reminded that medicine is a constantly evolving science and while the authors and publishers have ensured that all dosages, applications and practices are based on current indications, there may be specific practices which differ between communities. You should always follow the guidelines laid down by the manufacturers of specific products and the relevant authorities in the country in which you are practising.

Although every effort has been made to ensure that all owners of copyright material have been acknowledged in this publication, we would be pleased to acknowledge in subsequent reprints or editions any omissions brought to our attention.

Registered names, trademarks, etc. used in this book, even when not marked as such, are not to be considered unprotected by law.

Typeset by Medlar Publishing Solutions Pvt Ltd, India
Cover design by Andrew Magee Design
Printed in the UK

Last digit is the print number: 10 9 8 7 6 5 4 3 2 1

Contents

Preface

During the 20 years I have spent working within Rheumatology as a Clinician and Researcher, the specialty has undergone rapid changes. In many conditions this has led to earlier diagnosis and treatment of diseases which span this multisystem discipline of medicine.

As a teacher and trainer, I was approached by medical students, doctors-in-training, nurses, pharmacists, physiotherapists and occupational therapists, who attended my lectures at St George's, University of London. They all expressed a desire to understand the multidisciplinary management of patients living with rheumatological conditions through worked examples. Learners are often overwhelmed by the diagnostic criteria for rheumatic conditions, many of which have recently undergone review. In addition, the huge growth in disease-modifying therapies, including synthetic disease-modifying antirheumatic drugs (DMARDs) and biologic drugs can seem daunting to learners new to the field.

To address the unmet need of providing up-to-date summaries of clinical diagnosis and management of the most common rheumatic conditions, I have written this book with my co-authors, Zoe Rutter-Locher, a trainee in Rheumatology, and Helen Oakley, a physiotherapist working in Musculoskeletal Medicine. Zoe's input has been invaluable in identifying the questions that trainees who are new to Rheumatology are likely to ask. Helen's input as a physiotherapist has been crucial in explaining physiotherapy's contribution to the multidisciplinary components of care that many patients with rheumatic conditions require.

The book is divided into chapters which discuss each of the common rheumatological conditions, their diagnosis, the most up-to-date diagnostic criteria and management, based on UK NICE (National Institute of Health and Care Excellence) guidelines.

Assessment is an important part of learning, so each chapter also includes case histories discussing diagnosis and management, with discussion of answers provided for each case. References for NICE guidelines and further reading are also provided where appropriate.

Finally, I would like to say that this book is intended to provide a practical guide and aide memoire, which can be carried on ward rounds, in clinics and GP surgeries, to provide a concise summary of rheumatological conditions and their management.

I dedicate this book to all our patients whom we are here to serve.

Professor Nidhi Sofat
Professor of Rheumatology
St George's, University of London

Abbreviations

A&E	Accident and Emergency
ACR	American College of Rheumatology
ALT	alanine transaminase
ANA	antinuclear antibody
ANCA	anti-neutrophil cytoplasmic antibody
ARMA	Arthritis and Musculoskeletal Alliance
AS	ankylosing spondylitis
ASAS	Assessment of SpondyloArthritis international Society
AST	aspartate aminotransferase
BASDAI	Bath Ankylosing Spondylitis Disease Activity Index
BESS	British Elbow & Shoulder Society
BMD	bone mineral density
BMI	body mass index
BML	bone marrow lesion
BNF	British National Formulary
BNP	brain natriuretic peptide
BSR	British Society of Rheumatology
CBT	cognitive behavioural therapy
CK	creatine kinase
CMC	carpometacarpal
CPGS	Chronic Pain Grade Scale
CPP	calcium pyrophosphate

CPPD	calcium pyrophosphate deposition disease
CRP	C-reactive protein
CRPS	complex regional pain syndrome
CT	computerised tomography
CXR	chest X-ray
DAS	Disease Activity Score
DEXA	dual energy X-ray absorptiometry
DLCO	diffuse capacity of the lungs for carbon monoxide
DMARD	disease-modifying antirheumatic drug
dsDNA	double-stranded DNA
ECG	electrocardiogram
ED	emergency department
eGFR	estimated glomerular filtration rate
EGPA	eosinophilic granulomatosis with polyangiitis
ELISA	enzyme-linked immunosorbent assay
EMG	electromyography
ESR	erythrocyte sedimentation rate
EULAR	European League Against Rheumatism
FBC	full blood count
FDA	Food and Drugs Administration
FRAX	fracture risk algorithm
GCA	giant cell arteritis
GI	gastrointestinal
GP	general practitioner
GRACE index	GRAppa Composite score index
GWAS	genome-wide association studies
HEp-2	human epithelial type 2
HGPRT	hypoxanthine-guanine phosphoribosyltransferase
HIV	human immunodeficiency virus
HRCT	high resolution computerised tomography
IA	intra-articular

IIM	idiopathic inflammatory myopathies
ILD	interstitial lung disease
IM	intramuscular
IV	intravenous
JAK	Janus kinase
JIA	juvenile idiopathic arthritis
LDH	lactate dehydrogenase
LFTs	liver function tests
MALT	mucosa-associated lymphoid tissue
MAS	macrophage activation syndrome
MCP	metacarpophalangeal
MDT	multidisciplinary team
MGUS	multiple myeloma undetermined significance
MHC	major histocompatibility complex
MPO	myeloperoxidase
MS	multiple sclerosis
MSU	monosodium urate
MTP	metatarsophalangeal
NASS	National Axial Spondyloarthritis Society
NICE	National Institute for Health and Care Excellence
NSAID	non-steroidal anti-inflammatory drug
NSIP	non-specific interstitial pneumonia
OA	osteoarthritis
PAH	pulmonary arterial hypertension
PASDAS	Psoriatic ArthritiS Disease Activity Score
PASI	Psoriasis Area and Severity Index
PET	positron emission tomography
PIP	proximal interphalangeal
PMP	pain management programme
PO	per os (by mouth)

PPI	proton pump inhibitor
PRP	platelet-rich plasma
PRPP	phosphoribosyl pyrophosphate
PsA	psoriatic arthritis
PsARC	Psoriatic Arthritis Response Criteria
PTH	parathyroid hormone
RA	rheumatoid arthritis
RANK	receptor activator of nuclear factor kappa-B
RhF	rheumatoid factor
RS3PE	remitting seronegative symmetrical synovitis with pitting oedema
SC	subcutaneous
SLE	systemic lupus erythematosus
SNRI	serotonin–noradrenaline reuptake inhibitor
SSRI	selective serotonin reuptake inhibitor
STIR	short T1 inversion recovery
SUA	serum uric acid
TB	tuberculosis
TCA	tricyclic antidepressant
TLR	toll-like receptors
TNF	tumour necrosis factor
TRPV	transient potential receptor vanilloid
TSH	thyroid-stimulating hormone
U+Es	urea and electrolytes
UIP	usual interstitial pneumonia
ULT	urate-lowering therapy
US	ultrasound
VAS	Visual Analog Scale

C H A P T E R   1

Rheumatoid arthritis

1.1 Introduction

Rheumatoid arthritis (RA) is the archetypal autoimmune disease, demonstrating activation of several inflammatory pathways that, without early treatment, results in end-organ damage focused around synovial joints. Since RA is a systemic disease, other organs can also be involved, including the lungs, heart, eyes and central nervous system. The condition has a worldwide prevalence of 1–2%. RA affects women 2–3 times more often than men. Although RA can present at any age, patients most commonly are first affected in the third to sixth decades of life.

In this chapter we discuss the diagnosis, pathophysiology and management of RA in the context of real-life clinical cases. The cases aim to demonstrate the breadth of clinical scenarios in which RA can present, with worked examples of diagnosis and management, particularly in the context of biologic therapies, which have revolutionised RA care worldwide.

1.2 Diagnosis

The diagnosis of RA has been aided by the development of classification criteria published in 2010 (EULAR/ACR criteria, see Aletaha *et al.*, 2010). These include features that assist in confirming a diagnosis which is likely to require treatment (summarised in *Figure 1.1*). The features are based on:
- the pattern of joint involvement (joint distribution scores 0–5)
- the presence of autoantibodies (serology scores 0–3)

a	Parameter	Score
	Joint distribution (0–5)	
	1 large joint	0
	2–10 large joints	1
	1–3 small joints (large joints not counted)	2
	4–10 small joints (large joints not counted)	3
	>10 joints (at least one small joint)	5
	Serology (0–3)	
	Negative RA <u>and</u> negative ACPA	0
	Low positive RhF <u>or</u> low positive ACPA	2
	High positive RhF <u>or</u> high positive ACPA	3
	Symptom duration (0–1)	
	<6 weeks	0
	>6 weeks	1
	Acute phase reactants	
	Normal CRP <u>and</u> normal ESR	0
	Abnormal CRP <u>or</u> abnormal ESR	1
	Total >6 definite RA	

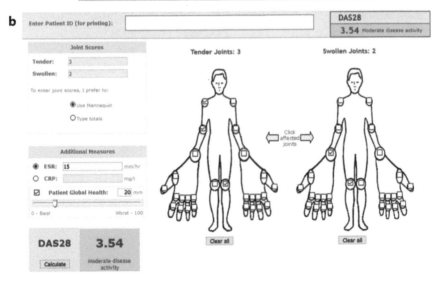

Figure 1.1. EULAR/ACR classification and DAS28 scoring system
(a) EULAR/ACR 2010 classification criteria for rheumatoid arthritis; (b) DAS28 scoring system – a freely available online tool that can be used in the clinic to calculate the Disease Activity Score (DAS) based on 28 joints assessed clinically for swelling and tenderness (see www.4s-dawn.com/DAS28). Scores are entered in the tool, together with inflammatory markers ESR or CRP, with the patient global assessment of their disease on a 0–100mm scale. A numerical DAS28 score is then calculated and recorded.

- the duration of symptoms, with >6 weeks' duration of symptoms making the diagnosis more likely (symptom duration scores 0–1)
- the presence of raised inflammatory markers, including erythrocyte sedimentation rate (ESR) and C-reactive protein (CRP) (acute phase reactants scores 0–1).

Depending on the presence/absence of such classification criteria, the criteria define a score. The higher the score, the greater the likelihood of confirming RA which is likely to require treatment intervention to achieve symptom control; a score >6 means a definite diagnosis of RA.

Prominent features of RA in comparison to osteoarthritis include the diurnal variation of symptoms, with prominent early morning stiffness, joint swelling due to synovitis in a symmetrical distribution in the small joints of the hand, and evidence of a systemic inflammatory response measured on blood tests including CRP and ESR.

In the early stages of disease, plain X-rays of the hands and feet are often performed to assess the presence of erosions or osteopenia, which can be monitored with treatment. In addition, ultrasound or MRI may be helpful in confirming the clinical findings of joint swelling, including synovitis or early erosions, which are indicators of joint damage that is likely to require early intervention.

1.3 Causes

RA is an autoimmune condition that is characterised by the presence of autoantibodies to rheumatoid factor (RhF) and anti-citrullinated (anti-CCP or ACPA) antibodies. The presence of these antibodies often predates the development of RA joint features by many years.

The development of RA is believed to be a multistep process (*Figure 1.2*):
- a genetic background such as the presence of susceptibility genes including alleles of the major histocompatibility complex (MHC) genes e.g. HLA-DR4, HLA-DR and PTPN22
- epigenetic factors such as the presence of autoantibodies
- associated environmental risks such as periodontal disease and smoking.

3

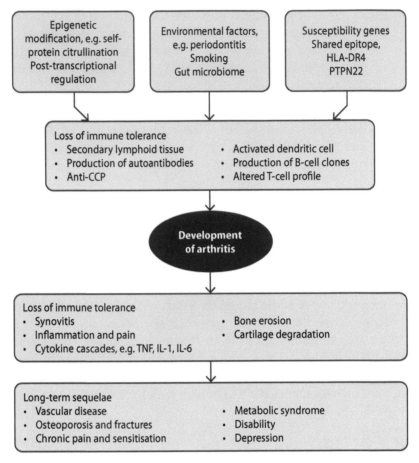

Figure 1.2. The development of rheumatoid arthritis

The factors described above all raise the likelihood of developing RA.

RA often develops as a systemic disease (meaning that it can affect the whole body) with the loss of immune tolerance, ongoing production of autoantibodies, proliferation of lymphoid tissue and activation of dendritic cells. Stimulation of the adaptive immune system leads to activation of several proinflammatory pathways, with initiation of cytokine cascades leading to changes focused around joints that include synovitis, bone erosions, inflammation and pain.

Because RA is a multisystem autoimmune condition, many changes occur including vascular inflammation, pain, inflammation, osteoporosis and metabolic changes, which can lead to extra-articular involvement.

1.4 Management

Once the diagnosis has been established, care is based on rapid suppression of inflammation and pain based on the concept of 'treat-to-target'.

1.4.1 Non-pharmacological management

There is evidence supporting the role of early exercise therapy in RA, including for example hand therapy to strengthen and maintain muscles, tendons and ligaments, and physiotherapy. Exercise is recommended, including physiotherapy, hand therapy and occupational therapy (NICE guideline [NG100] Published date: July 2018).

1.4.2 Pharmacological management

One of the early features of RA is pain and therefore pain management is a cornerstone of early treatment. Trial evidence shows that non-steroidal anti-inflammatory drugs (NSAIDs) are key to control early pain and inflammation. NICE guidance states that NSAIDs should be prescribed at the lowest dose possible for the shortest period of time in RA, ensuring that cardiovascular, renal and gastrointestinal risk factors are considered on a patient-by-patient basis (https://cks.nice.org.uk/nsaids-prescribing-issues#!scenario). NICE also recommends that gastroprotection in the form of a proton pump inhibitor (PPI) is cost-effective in people with conditions such as RA. In cases where several risk factors exist, e.g. cardiovascular, gastrointestinal in elderly patients, topical NSAIDs can be considered.

First-line therapy

First-line therapy in the treat-to-target regimen is considered to be oral synthetic disease-modifying antirheumatic drugs (DMARDs), including methotrexate, sulfasalazine, leflunomide and hydroxychloroquine. If the patient has not achieved their treat-to-target DAS28 within the first 3–6 months of synthetic DMARD therapy, they can be considered for second-line biologic therapies.

Disease-modifying antirheumatic drugs

In recent years, the concept of treat-to-target has been developed to guide treatment for RA (NICE guideline [NG100] Published date: July 2018). Treatment regimens are developed based on the level of disease activity score (DAS28).

The use of DMARDs has been widely adopted in clinical guidelines internationally. The current agents used as first- and second-line therapy are summarised in *Table 1.1*. Evidence shows that the earlier control of inflammation and pain is achieved, the more likely the patient is to be free of long-term sequelae including joint damage, functional loss and co-morbidities such as osteoporosis and vascular disease. There is therefore a good rationale for early diagnosis of RA, initiation of early DMARD therapy with subsequent monitoring that improves long-term outcomes and survival.

In the clinic, with the availability of a wide range of new therapies, the challenge for the clinician is to ensure the patient is counselled and selected for the right treatment at the right time. The approach most commonly used is:

- First-line – therapy with conventional synthetic DMARDs, e.g. methotrexate, sulfasalazine or hydroxychloroquine. Typically the treat-to-target DAS28 score will be 3.5–4.5
- Second-line – therapies such as tumour necrosis factor (TNF) inhibitors, B-cell depletion and other biologic immunotherapies are added if treat-to-target DAS28 score of >5.1 is reached
- NICE guidelines (2018, NG100) state that if patients are not achieving their target DAS28, then escalation therapy can be initiated. Typically, a sustained DAS28 score of >5.1, suggesting uncontrolled high disease activity, warrants initiation of biologic DMARDs including NICE-approved medications such as adalimumab, etanercept, certolizumab pegol, golimumab, tocilizumab and abatacept.

Biologic therapies

Biologic therapies are considered to be second-line therapies in the treat-to-target scheme (NICE, 2018, NG100). In the last two decades, effective biologic drugs have been developed which have significantly improved outcomes for patients and have led to

Table 1.1. Most commonly used agents for rheumatoid arthritis according to UK guidelines (rows with light background are synthetic DMARDs; those with darker background are biologic DMARDs)

Drug	Formulation and dose	Mechanism of action	Usual level of therapy (NICE guidelines)	Screening	Monitoring
Methotrexate	PO/SC Typically 15–25mg weekly	Inhibition of purine synthesis	1st line	Hepatitis B & C, HIV	FBC, U+Es, LFTs
Leflunomide	PO Typically 20mg daily after loading dose	Inhibition of pyrimidine synthesis	1st line	Hepatitis B & C, HIV	FBC, U+Es, LFTs
Azathioprine	PO Typically 50–150mg daily in divided doses	Inhibition of purine synthesis	1st line	Hepatitis B & C, HIV	FBC, U+Es, LFTs
Sulfasalazine	PO Typically 1–3g daily in divided doses	Inhibitor of expression of TNF and other cytokines	1st line	Hepatitis B & C, HIV	FBC, U+Es, LFTs
Hydroxychloroquine	PO Up to 400mg daily in divided doses	Inhibitor of expression of TNF and other cytokines	1st line	Hepatitis B & C, HIV	FBC, U+Es, LFTs
Corticosteroids, e.g. prednisolone	PO/IM Typically 120–180mg IM Range 15–40mg oral daily on reducing dose	Works through multiple pathways including increased transcription of anti-inflammatory genes	1st line	Monitor for diabetes, hypertension	
Infliximab (Remicade/Remsima biosimilar)	IV 0-, 2-, 6- then 8-weekly at 5mg/kg	Chimeric anti-TNF monoclonal antibody	2nd line	Hepatitis B & C, HIV	FBC, U+Es, LFTs
Adalimumab (Humira)	40mg SC every 2 weeks	Humanised anti-TNF monoclonal antibody	2nd line	Hepatitis B & C, HIV	FBC, U+Es, LFTs
Etanercept (Enbrel, Benepali biosimilar)	50mg SC weekly or 25mg twice weekly	TNF receptor fusion protein	2nd line	Hepatitis B & C, HIV, TB	FBC, U+Es, LFTs

Table 1.1. (Continued)

Drug	Formulation and dose	Mechanism of action	Usual level of therapy (NICE guidelines)	Screening	Monitoring
Certolizumab	200mg every 2 weeks or 400mg every 4 weeks	Pegylated TNF antibody	2nd line	Hepatitis B & C, HIV, TB	FBC, U+Es, LFTs
Golimumab	50mg monthly Consider 100mg monthly on subjects >100kg if inadequate response at 50mg	Humanised anti-TNF monoclonal antibody	2nd line	Hepatitis B & C, HIV, TB	FBC, U+Es, LFTs
Tocilizumab (Actemra)	162mg SC weekly or 8mg/kg IV/SC every 4 weeks	Monoclonal antibody to IL-6 receptor	2nd line	Hepatitis B & C, HIV, TB	FBC, U+Es, LFTs, lipids
Sarilumab (Kevzara)	200mg SC every 2 weeks	Monoclonal antibody to IL-6 receptor	2nd line	Hepatitis B & C, HIV, TB	FBC, U+Es, LFTs, lipids
Anakinra	100mg SC daily	Interleukin-1 receptor antagonist fusion protein	2nd line	Hepatitis B & C, HIV	FBC, U+Es, LFTs
Abatacept (Orencia)	125mg SC weekly	Fusion protein of IgG1 and CTLA-4	2nd line	Hepatitis B & C, HIV, TB	FBC, U+Es, LFTs
Rituximab (Mabthera, Truxima biosimilar)	IV 1 g infusion 2 weeks apart then repeated after 6 months	Monoclonal antibody to CD20	2nd line	Hepatitis B & C, HIV, TB B-cell subsets	FBC, U+Es, LFTs
Baricitinib Tofacitinib	PO daily Baricitinib 2–4mg daily Tofacitinib 5mg twice daily	JAK inhibitors	2nd line	Hepatitis B & C, HIV, TB	FBC, U+Es, LFTs, lipids Monitor for herpes zoster

Abbreviations: FBC, full blood count; HIV, human immunodeficiency virus; IM, intramuscular; IV, intravenous; LFTs, liver function tests; PO, per os (by mouth); SC, subcutaneous; U+Es, urea and electrolytes.

incorporation of the treatments into UK NICE recommendations. The biologic treatments developed have evolved from a significantly improved understanding of the pathogenesis of RA, involving several immune pathways which mediate the joint damage and inflammation seen in people with RA. NICE recommends the management of RA with second-line biologics as step-up therapy when conventional synthetic DMARD therapies have not controlled disease activity. Biologic therapies are targeted at specific cytokines, including adalimumab, etanercept, infliximab, certolizumab pegol, golimumab, rituximab, sarilumab, tocilizumab, abatacept, baricitinib and tofacitinib. The number of licensed biologic therapies available continues to grow.

Cytokines

Cytokines, including tumour necrosis factor alpha (TNF-α) and IL-6, are involved in mediating the pathogenesis of RA. Examples of highly specific antibody-based therapies targeted at selective cytokine inhibition include the following:
- Monoclonals targeted at TNF-α: adalimumab, etanercept, infliximab, certolizumab pegol, golimumab
- Monoclonals targeted at IL-6: sarilumab, tocilizumab.

Current guidance recommends using the most cost-effective therapy after assessing patients for appropriate therapies. For example, TNF inhibitors are not used in subjects with a history of cancer within the last 5 years, serious infections requiring long-term antibiotics, a history of multiple sclerosis, or uncontrolled ischaemic heart disease/cardiac failure. In such cases, an alternative biologic agent to TNF inhibitors may be required, e.g. B cell-based therapies.

B-cell blockers and other therapies

Inhibition of distinct pathways of the immune system, including depletion of B cells (with B-cell depletion therapy) or co-stimulatory molecules (CTLA 4), have also been shown to be effective therapies in RA. Most recently, clinical trials with Janus kinase (JAK) inhibitors have shown that cytokine receptors which signal through JAK/STAT pathway are important in RA.

Immunisations in people on DMARD therapies

It is usually recommended that patients should have live vaccines before they start their DMARD therapy, e.g. yellow fever. Vaccines which have attenuated or killed antigen, e.g. pneumovax, are also recommended. Subjects on DMARDs are also advised to have the annual influenza vaccination.

1.5 Cases

The following case histories are real-life examples demonstrating diagnosis and decision-making processes for RA management in the context of conventional and biologic therapies available for treatment.

Case history 1.1

A 28-year-old woman presented to her GP with acute onset pain and stiffness in her hands and body for the last 3 months. She had her first child with a normal delivery 10 months previously and was struggling to cope. Her GP had prescribed ibuprofen 200mg TDS and arranged blood tests, which showed:
- ESR 78mm/h
- CRP 56g/L
- Anti-CCP antibodies 156
- Rheumatoid factor 46

She was referred urgently to a rheumatologist. On assessment in the rheumatology clinic, a diagnosis of acute seropositive rheumatoid arthritis was made, based on the history, investigations and physical signs of synovitis in her metacarpophalangeal joints and wrists. She did not have plans to have another child in the near future.

What treatment would you recommend?

A range of options are available:
- Anti-TNF monoclonal antibody
- Intramuscular Depo-Medrone
- Methotrexate and hydroxychloroquine
- Methotrexate, leflunomide and hydroxychloroquine
- Oral steroid-weaning regime and methotrexate

For this patient, the most appropriate treatment is oral steroid (on a weaning regime) and methotrexate. Corticosteroids are very effective at suppressing pain and inflammation rapidly and are therefore commonly used in the early stages of RA or during flare-ups. However, when used long-term, corticosteroids have significant side-effects, including weight gain, skin thinning, diabetes mellitus and hypertension. In the context of RA treatment, corticosteroids should only be used for short periods and long-term therapy in the form of DMARDs. It is better to use steroids for short periods, e.g. to control disease flares or to suppress inflammation at acute presentation, in order to avoid the development of long-term steroid-related side-effects including weight gain, Cushingoid features, thin skin, easy bruising, impaired glucose tolerance and/or diabetes, osteoporosis and infection risk.

The patient was commenced on a course of corticosteroids, starting with prednisolone 20mg per day, on a dose reducing by 5mg every week. The aim of this type of steroid dosing is to reduce the joint inflammation caused by synovitis that leads to acute swelling, pain and stiffness, often in a symmetrical distribution in the small joints of the hands, wrists, elbows and knees.

The initiation of longer-term DMARD therapy was also discussed with the patient. Current NICE recommendations discuss initiation of therapy early to prevent long-term damage to the joints, to 'switch off' inflammation, and to prevent the longer-term effects of sustained inflammation, including hypertension, osteoporosis and muscle wasting. The concept of 'treat-to-target' has shown that setting a target for treatment, and then instituting treatment including oral and/or biologic DMARDs to achieve remission, achieves better outcomes long-term in RA.

After discussing the pros and cons of different DMARD therapies (see *Table 1.1*), the patient decided to proceed with methotrexate therapy of 20mg at a weekly dose, also taking folic acid 5mg one day after methotrexate.

You see her again in two weeks and she is experiencing side-effects, with severe nausea on the day of taking methotrexate.

What option is best to help with the nausea?

- Increase folic acid to 5mg three times a week
- Prescribe an antiemetic
- Reduce dose of methotrexate to 15mg weekly
- Switch methotrexate to hydroxychloroquine
- Tell her there is nothing you can do

Nausea and mouth ulcers can both be helped by increasing the folic acid dose either to 10mg on the day of administration or by increasing the frequency (patients should be reminded not to take folic acid on the same day as the methotrexate). This patient has active disease and so if possible the best course of action is to remain on methotrexate at the dose of 20mg weekly in order to induce remission of disease.

Four months after starting therapy, the patient went into remission and did not require any further steroid or NSAID and was only on oral methotrexate DMARD therapy treatment. She continues to be reviewed on a 6-monthly basis in the rheumatology clinic.

How do we define remission according to DAS28?

A DAS28 score of <2.6 is generally accepted to be a score demonstrating good disease control.

All patients with RA who are attending a rheumatology clinic should have their disease activity score measured. The most widely accepted score of disease activity is the disease activity score based on assessment of the 28 most commonly affected joints (see *Figure 1.1* and www.4s-dawn.com/DAS28/ for further information). An assessment is made by the clinician of the tender joint count and swollen joint count from the joints assessed. This score, combined with the ESR or CRP, plus the patient global assessment of their disease activity (on a scale of 0–100mm) provides a score which is practical to measure in the clinic and can be used to evaluate response to therapy. The clinical value of a DAS28 score includes repeat scoring after instituting a new DMARD therapy in order to 'treat-to-target' to induce clinical remission.

Tight disease control is associated with improved outcomes for patients. For example, the TICORA study found that patients who underwent intensive outpatient management using predefined goals to standard care had reduced disease activity, radiographic disease progression, and improved physical function and quality of life at no additional cost.

If the patient says that she is considering having a second child, what advice regarding her medications would you give her?

· Continue methotrexate
· Stop methotrexate 3m prior to conception
· Stop methotrexate 6m prior to conception
· Switch to anti-TNF
· Switch to leflunomide

Methotrexate and leflunomide have a risk of fetal malformations and teratogenicity, especially when taken by the pregnant mother in the first trimester of pregnancy, and so you should advise the patient to stop taking the methotrexate 3 months before conception.

A group of drugs for which the manufacturers urge caution, but with lower risk of fetal malformations, includes the DMARDs sulfasalazine, azathioprine and hydroxychloroquine.

Biologics, including TNF-α inhibitors, have generally been found to be safe in pregnancy in several international studies, but the British Society for Rheumatology guidelines advise stopping anti-TNF at different stages of pregnancy, with tocilizumab and rituximab stopped prior to conception (Flint *et al.*, 2016). All women and men on DMARD therapies should be counselled about using contraception while they are on DMARD therapy to prevent fetal problems.

Case history 1.2

A 36-year-old lady with seropositive RA has been attending the rheumatology clinic for the last 6 years. She recently gave birth to her third child and now comes to clinic with her 4-month-old baby. During her pregnancy, she stopped all DMARD therapy, which had included methotrexate and hydroxychloroquine. She had taken a few courses of oral prednisolone during pregnancy for joint flares.

In clinic she has acute pain in her right thumb. She is unable to abduct or rotate her thumb. You suspect an acute rupture of the abductor pollicis longus tendon. After contacting the hand surgeon, the diagnosis is confirmed and she undergoes urgent tendon repair.

Four weeks later, she is reviewed in the rheumatology clinic. Her joints have flared again, she is finding it difficult to hold her baby, and her DAS28 score is 5.8.

What treatment do you think is most appropriate to offer her?

- Anti-TNF monoclonal antibody
- Hydroxychloroquine
- Methotrexate and hydroxychloroquine
- Rituximab
- Tocilizumab

It is well known that RA can flare following pregnancy and so it is most appropriate for the patient to go back on methotrexate and hydroxychloroquine. She agrees after you explain that stopping her DMARDs in pregnancy left her RA less well controlled. She would not yet be eligible for biologic therapy as per NICE guidance which requires "DAS28 score >5.1 and disease has not responded to intensive therapy with a combination of at least 2 conventional DMARDs".

She is also prescribed a course of prednisolone to treat her acute wrist and metacarpophalangeal (MCP) swelling as the methotrexate and hydroxychloroquine are likely to take 6–8 weeks to work. The patient is advised not to breastfeed as she has now restarted methotrexate. Follow-up is arranged in 3 months.

The patient is reviewed in 3 months but continues to have ongoing early morning stiffness lasting a few hours each day, and clinically has active disease with a DAS28 score of 5.6.

What treatment plan would you discuss?

Treatment escalation in the form of biologic DMARDs should be discussed because the patient continues to have active disease with a DAS28 score >5.1 despite the use of two conventional DMARDs. She is counselled and agrees to initiate adalimumab therapy.

What screening does the patient need to have before starting TNF inhibitor therapy?

The patient should be screened for any previous history of cancer, severe infections, history or family history of multiple sclerosis, or history of tuberculosis (TB).

The patient reports that her mother may have had TB. She undergoes TB screening with a Mantoux test, which is weak positive after 48h, and she has a negative Quantiferon test. In view of her possible previous exposure to TB, with the Mantoux test result, she is given 3 months of TB prophylaxis treatment before initiating TNF inhibitor therapy. Six months after starting TNF inhibitor treatment, in combination with methotrexate and hydroxychloroquine, she has a DAS28 score of 3.6 and continues with this therapy.

Case history 1.3

A 57-year-old man with seropositive RA is an outpatient at the rheumatology clinic. He has been treated with methotrexate for the last 2 years and has been in remission. Over the last few months he has developed increasing shortness of breath and a non-productive cough.

He visits his GP surgery about the shortness of breath and a chest radiograph is performed in the GP surgery. The GP refers him urgently to rheumatology; lung function tests and a high resolution computerised tomography (HRCT) scan of the chest (see below) are arranged. The CT scan shows patchy NSIP (non-specific interstitial pneumonia), which is described with RA.

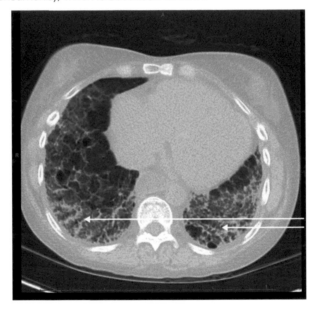

Arrows in figure show ground glass changes.

What pattern would you expect to see on CT images?

- Bronchial wall thickening and signet ring sign
- Bullae
- Ground glass subpleural changes
- Honeycombing with lung architecture distortion
- Multiple pulmonary nodules

It is usual for ground glass subpleural changes to be visible. RA interstitial lung disease (RA-ILD) is a rare but important extra-articular manifestation of RA because it is associated with significant morbidity and mortality. Diagnosis is based on HRCT findings and pulmonary function tests which typically indicate a fibrotic pattern with restrictive physiology and reduced diffusing capacity. Risk factors for its development include male gender, a smoking history and long-standing RA. Based on the pattern of distribution, the fibrotic changes are classified into UIP (usual interstitial pneumonia) and NSIP (non-specific interstitial pneumonia).

What changes would you make to his treatment?

Because methotrexate can cause pulmonary fibrosis in a patient who has been on this medication for some time, it is difficult to know at which stage the changes developed. Following discussion in the lung multidisciplinary team (MDT) meeting, the methotrexate is stopped and he is switched to mycophenolate mofetil (an immunosuppressant).

He tolerates the drug, maintains his lung function and his arthritis is controlled. Another medication which is used in the setting of RA-related lung fibrosis is rituximab therapy.

Case history 1.4

A 46-year-old male has been treated for seropositive RA for the last 18 years. He has responded originally to methotrexate, followed by infliximab. He stopped responding to infliximab after 4 years and so was switched to etanercept. Three months after starting etanercept, he developed an acute skin hypersensitivity reaction and the etanercept was stopped. He was then started on 6-monthly infusions of rituximab, which worked for 2 years. He then developed severe pneumonia and flared in his joints. A repeat rituximab infusion failed to control his symptoms. He was then switched to the JAK inhibitor, baricitinib. Five months after initiating therapy, he is in remission.

When should Janus kinase inhibitors be used?

JAK inhibitors, including tofacitinib and baricitinib, are relatively new agents that have been introduced for the management of active RA, particularly when second-line therapy in the form of TNF inhibitors has been unsuccessful. As with TNF inhibitors, patients need to have close blood monitoring and be screened for infection risk before and during treatment. JAK inhibitors have a shorter half-life than TNF inhibitors and are taken orally. They are also associated with potential infection risk, and all patients should be warned of this. In the case of tofacitinib, a higher rate of viral infections has been noted than with TNF inhibitors.

Case history 1.5

A 26-year-old lady is referred to the rheumatology clinic with joint pains. An autoantibody check reveals that she is strongly CCP antibody positive, but she has a normal ESR and CRP, and clinically there is no joint inflammation including synovitis.

What advice should the patient be given?

It is a relatively common clinical scenario to present with polyarthralgia when CCP antibodies are found to be positive but there is no active synovitis. European League Against Rheumatism (EULAR) and American College of Rheumatology (ACR) criteria state that inflammatory features of synovitis of >6 weeks are required for treatment to be initiated. In cases such as these, it is best to monitor the patient, e.g. every 6 months, to observe if they progress to synovitis. If they do, then DMARD therapy can be offered, but patients may not develop synovitis and in those cases would not require initiation of DMARD therapy.

Case history 1.6

A 76-year-old lady presents to Accident and Emergency (A&E) because she is very weak and has developed joint pains in her hands and arms with acute swelling in her hands. She reports that the same symptoms occurred a few months previously and improved with NSAIDs, but this time the symptoms were more severe and not controlled with NSAIDs. On assessment, the doctor finds pitting oedema in both hands and queries cellulitis. However, in view of the joint pain, the rheumatology team are asked to assess the patient and evidence of synovitis is found in the small joints of the hands.

What is the most likely diagnosis?

- Cellulitis
- Rheumatoid arthritis
- Osteoarthritis
- Allergic reaction
- Remitting seronegative symmetrical synovitis with pitting oedema (RS3PE) syndrome

Based on the history, remitting seronegative symmetrical synovitis with pitting oedema (RS3PE) syndrome is more likely than cellulitis. RS3PE syndrome is a rare condition which causes a symmetrical polyarthritis, synovitis and acute pitting oedema of the dorsum of the hands and/or feet. It is typified by a negative serum RhF or CCP antibodies. In the context of no other underlying diagnoses, idiopathic RS3PE syndrome is a rare but important condition to diagnose because it is associated with good response to treatments with low-dose corticosteroids. Typically, a dose ranging between 15 and 20mg daily of prednisolone (the preferred corticosteroid) is effective in treating this condition, with dose-tapering over 3–6 months.

Case history 1.7

A 60-year-old man with rheumatoid arthritis comes to the emergency department (ED). He has developed acute onset pain and swelling in his right knee. His RA is usually well controlled on oral weekly methotrexate. He has been gardening and was bitten on his leg by an insect a few days ago. On examination, he has a temperature of 38.1°C. He is finding it difficult to bend his knee, which is red and swollen. The ED doctor aspirates the knee to obtain 12ml of yellow thick liquid. The synovial fluid is sent for urgent Gram stain and culture. The urgent Gram stain shows Gram-positive cocci.

What is the most likely diagnosis?

· Streptococcal septic arthritis
· Tuberculous infection
· Viral infection
· Flare of rheumatoid arthritis
· Traumatic knee effusion

With the history and clinical presentation, and evidence of Gram-positive cocci on synovial fluid aspiration, the diagnosis is a septic arthritis in a patient with rheumatoid arthritis who is on immune-modulatory treatment. He is started on intravenous flucloxacillin and his condition improves within a few days. He requires a prolonged course of antibiotics for 6 weeks and remains off methotrexate until his septic arthritis improves.

Case history 1.8

A 36-year-old man presented to A&E with polyarthralgia and shortness of breath. He was on holiday in Spain 2 months ago when he developed a sore throat, cough and diarrhoea for a few days. His symptoms improved after a week. His joint pains and breathlessness developed 3 days ago. He was unable to wash and dress himself and noticed fevers at night.

The doctor in A&E found evidence of an inflammatory arthritis on clinical examination with a symmetrical polyarthropathy of both hands. He also had dullness to percussion at both lung bases with bilateral pleural effusions confirmed on chest radiography.

An infection screen was performed including blood cultures, QuantiFERON test for tuberculosis, hepatitis B/C and HIV serology, all of which were negative.
- ESR 79mm/h
- CRP 87mg/L
- Anti-CCP antibodies 3
- Rheumatoid factor negative
- ANA negative
- Ferritin 3450 mcg/L

He also has a CT chest, abdomen and pelvis which showed mediastinal and axillary lymphadenopathy with bilateral pleural effusions, but no evidence of malignancy. Lymph node biopsy showed reactive lymph nodes and no malignancy.

What is the most likely diagnosis?

- Seronegative rheumatoid arthritis
- Parvovirus infection
- Adult onset Still's disease
- Lymphoma
- Rheumatic fever

The most likely diagnosis is adult onset Still's disease. The patient had a negative infection screen, normal lymph node biopsy and negative autoantibodies. Adult onset Still's disease is often typified by fevers, polyarthralgia, rashes and serositis. Patients can develop an inflammatory arthritis. Rashes, typically a salmon-pink rash, coincide with the fever. The patient responded to oral corticosteroid therapy in the form of prednisolone starting at 30mg daily on a reducing dose, followed by hydroxychloroquine DMARD therapy to control his joint symptoms. He remained in remission at one year and his inflammatory markers returned to normal.

1.6 References

Aletaha, D., Neogi, T., Silman, A.J. *et al.* (2010) Rheumatoid arthritis classification criteria. *Arthritis and Rheumatology*, **62**: 2569.

Flint, J., Panchal, S., Hurrell, A. *et al.* (2016) BSR and BHPR guideline on prescribing drugs in pregnancy and breastfeeding—Part I: standard and biologic disease modifying anti-rheumatic drugs and corticosteroids. *Rheumatology*, **55**: 1693.

Grigor, C., Capell, H., Sirling, A. *et al.* (2004) Effect of a treatment strategy of tight control for rheumatoid arthritis (the TICORA study): a single blind randomised controlled trial. *Lancet*, **364(9340)**: 263–9.

McInnes, I.B. and Schett, G. (2017) Pathogenetic insights from the treatment of rheumatoid arthritis. *Lancet*, 10; **389(10086)**: 2328–2337.

Smolen, J.S., Aletaha, D., Barton, A. *et al.* (2018) Rheumatoid arthritis. *Nature Reviews Disease Primers*, **4:** 18001. doi: 10.1038/nrdp.2018.1.

Smolen, J.S., Landewe, R., Bijlsma, J. *et al.* (2017) EULAR recommendations for the management of rheumatoid arthritis with synthetic and biological disease-modifying antirheumatic drugs: 2016 update. *Ann Rheum Dis.*, **76**: 960–977.

NICE, BSR guidelines and useful websites

NICE guidelines for the management of RA (2018, NG100)
www.nice.org.uk/guidance/ng100

www.nras.org.uk/the-role-of-the-physiotherapist-in-rheumatoid-arthritis

British Society for Rheumatology Guidelines for monitoring

www.rheumatology.org.uk/Knowledge/Excellence/Guidelines

(https://academic.oup.com/rheumatology/article/55/9/1693/1744535)

www.rheumatology.org.uk/practice-quality/guideline

Useful resources for classification of RA

Aletaha, D., Neogi, T., Silman, A.J. *et al.* (2010) 2010 rheumatoid arthritis classification criteria: an American College of Rheumatology/European League Against Rheumatism collaborative initiative. *Ann Rheum Dis.* **69(9)**: 1580–8.

Smolen, J.S., Aletaha, D., Bijlsma, J.W. *et al.* (2010) Treating rheumatoid arthritis to target: recommendations of an international task force. *Ann Rheum Dis.*, **69(4)**: 631–7.

Connective tissue disease

Connective tissue diseases are a heterogeneous spectrum of conditions including systemic lupus erythematosus (SLE), systemic sclerosis, myositis and Sjögren's syndrome, each presenting with typical features and autoimmune profiles. Often these conditions present with overlapping symptoms and they can be difficult to diagnose and perform clinical studies into. They are multisystem chronic conditions with complex aetiologies and pathogenesis, and so management must be aimed not only at the disease being treated, but also the severity of flare and organ which is involved.

This chapter will provide a brief overview of the diagnosis, pathophysiology and management of SLE, systemic sclerosis, myositis and Sjögren's syndrome, followed by a series of real-world cases in order to highlight more common clinical scenarios and work through diagnosis and management of these.

2.1 Systemic lupus erythematosus

2.1.1 Introduction

Systemic lupus erythematosus (SLE) is an autoimmune condition characterised by inflammation in many organ systems. The peak incidence of SLE is between 15 and 40 years of age. In this age group, women are 10 times more commonly affected than men. The predominance in female patients decreases with age. There are also racial differences in SLE prevalence: subjects of African and Asian descent often have a greater incidence of SLE and a tendency towards more severe disease. The overall prevalence of SLE in the population is approximately 25–50 per 100 000.

2.1.2 Diagnosis

SLE is an extremely heterogeneous disease, with a range of presentations from mild non-specific symptoms to severe life-threatening conditions. Symptoms and signs will not be present at all times and will change with flares in the disease. This makes diagnosis difficult and it must be made by an experienced clinician together with relevant investigations and careful consideration of alternative diagnoses.

Recently, approaches using clinician-based assessment and data-driven evaluation in combination have led to the publication of revised classification criteria for SLE (Aringer *et al.*, 2019). The new 2019 criteria supersede the 1997 ACR criteria and the 2012 SLICC (Systemic Lupus International Collaborating Clinics).

The 2019 EULAR/ACR classification criteria for SLE include a positive antinuclear antibody (ANA) measured at least once as a required entry criterion, followed by additional features which are grouped into seven clinical components, i.e. constitutional symptoms, haematological, neuropsychiatric, mucocutaneous, serosal, musculoskeletal and renal features (*Figure 2.1*). There are three immunological domains, which include antiphospholipid antibodies, complement proteins and SLE-specific antibodies. The individual components are weighted from 2–10. Subjects who accumulate 10 points or more are classified. The new criteria have a sensitivity of 96.1% and specificity of 96.7%, which is higher than previous criteria.

SLE presents with a wide range of clinical manifestations and can affect multiple organs. There are no pathognomonic features of SLE but it does tend to affect certain organs in typical patterns. The most typical clinical features of SLE can be divided into seven components:

- *Constitutional symptoms*: fever, weight loss, night sweats.
- *Haematological and lymphadenopathy*: lymphadenopathy is common and can increase during flares. Anaemia, lymphopenia and thrombocytopenia are also typical.
- *Neuropsychiatric*: lupus can present with a huge range of neurological and psychiatric symptoms including headaches, seizures, peripheral neuropathies, low mood and psychosis. Diagnosis is often difficult and alternative diagnoses must be excluded.
- *Mucocutaneous*: acute cutaneous lupus erythematosus including classic 'butterfly' rash, which is a fixed photosensitive erythematous rash on the malar eminences and over the nose but sparing the nasolabial folds; subacute cutaneous lupus erythematosus which is a photosensitive rash, usually on sun-exposed areas and which can be papulosquamous or annular; classic discoid lupus is characterised by well demarcated and scaly plaques which leave central scars and changes in pigmentation.
- *Serosal*: pericarditis and valvular lesions can occur in SLE; typically, Libman–Sacks endocarditis occurs with deposition of thrombus vegetation. Myocardial involvement, however, is rare. Pleuritis is common, presenting with chest pains. Pulmonary involvement also includes acute pneumonitis, interstitial lung disease, pulmonary embolism, pleural effusions and pulmonary haemorrhage.
- *Musculoskeletal*: arthralgia affects about 90% of SLE patients. It can present with a non-erosive polyarthritis affecting the small joints of the hands. This can develop into Jaccoud arthropathy, a deformity which looks similar to rheumatoid arthritis with ulnar deviation, swan neck and boutonnière deformities, but is due to ligament laxity rather than bony erosions. Inflammatory myositis with proximal muscle weakness can sometimes occur.
- *Renal*: renal involvement in SLE is a major cause of morbidity and mortality. Although lupus nephritis can present with asymptomatic proteinuria, it is a potentially life-threatening form of SLE and regular monitoring with urine dipstick and protein:creatinine ratio must be performed. In cases where renal involvement is suspected, renal biopsy is usually performed to assess the stage of disease and plan treatment.

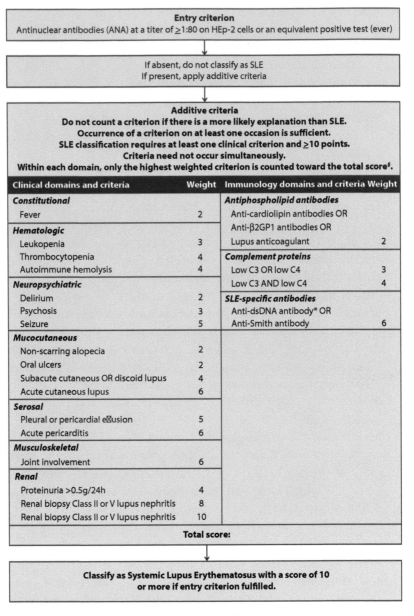

Entry criterion
Antinuclear antibodies (ANA) at a titer of $\geq$1:80 on HEp-2 cells or an equivalent positive test (ever)

If absent, do not classify as SLE
If present, apply additive criteria

Additive criteria
Do not count a criterion if there is a more likely explanation than SLE.
Occurrence of a criterion on at least one occasion is sufficient.
SLE classification requires at least one clinical criterion and $\geq$10 points.
Criteria need not occur simultaneously.
Within each domain, only the highest weighted criterion is counted toward the total score§.

Clinical domains and criteria	Weight	Immunology domains and criteria	Weight
Constitutional		**Antiphospholipid antibodies**	
Fever	2	Anti-cardiolipin antibodies OR	
Hematologic		Anti-β2GP1 antibodies OR	
Leukopenia	3	Lupus anticoagulant	2
Thrombocytopenia	4	**Complement proteins**	
Autoimmune hemolysis	4	Low C3 OR low C4	3
Neuropsychiatric		Low C3 AND low C4	4
Delirium	2	**SLE-specific antibodies**	
Psychosis	3	Anti-dsDNA antibody* OR	
Seizure	5	Anti-Smith antibody	6
Mucocutaneous			
Non-scarring alopecia	2		
Oral ulcers	2		
Subacute cutaneous OR discoid lupus	4		
Acute cutaneous lupus	6		
Serosal			
Pleural or pericardia! effusion	5		
Acute pericarditis	6		
Musculoskeletal			
Joint involvement	6		
Renal			
Proteinuria >0.5g/24h	4		
Renal biopsy Class II or V lupus nephritis	8		
Renal biopsy Class II or V lupus nephritis	10		
Total score:			

Classify as Systemic Lupus Erythematosus with a score of 10
or more if entry criterion fulfilled.

Figure 2.1. 2019 EULAR/ACR criteria for SLE
§Additional criteria items within the same domain will not be counted. *Note: in an assay with at least 90% specificity against relevant disease controls. Reproduced from Aringer, M., Costenbader, K., Daikh, D. *et al.* 2019 EULAR/ACR classification criteria for Systemic Lupus Erythematosus. *Ann Rheum Dis.*, 2019, **78**: 1151–9, with permission from BMJ Publishing Group Ltd.

Antibodies in SLE

Assessment of antibody status is recommended (see *Figure 2.1*). The most common antibodies used to assist in the diagnosis of SLE include the presence of a positive ANA at significant titre (>1:80) or on immunostaining of, for example, human epithelial type 2 (HEp-2) cells. In addition, the presence of anticardiolipin antibodies, anti-beta 2 glycoprotein antibodies or lupus anticoagulant, in combination with the clinical features described above, is used to assist in making a diagnosis of SLE. Other antibodies which are highly specific for SLE include the anti-double-stranded DNA antibody (dsDNA) and the anti-Smith antibody. Immunological measures of disease activity that are used to track disease activity and progression include the anti-dsDNA antibodies, together with complement C3 and C4 levels. High levels of anti-dsDNA antibodies suggest high disease activity, whereas low C3 and C4 levels also indicate high disease activity.

2.1.3 Causes

The aetiology and pathogenesis of SLE are complex. Individuals have a genetic predisposition and genome-wide association studies (GWAS) have identified multiple genes which increase the risk of developing SLE, albeit all to a small degree each. The condition only manifests as a result of environmental triggers, of which UV light, smoking, certain infections such as Epstein–Barr virus and drugs such as tetracyclines and hydralazine have been implicated. This leads to a breakdown in immune tolerance and stimulation of the immune response. The exact pathogenesis is not fully understood but there are important roles of defective clearance of apoptotic cells, activation of toll-like receptors (TLRs) and downstream signalling pathways, release of type 1 interferon and the activation of dysregulated B cells, leading to antibody production and immune complex deposition. Immune dysregulation leads to organ damage and the clinical features of SLE affecting different organ systems. The pathogenesis of SLE is summarised in *Figure 2.2*.

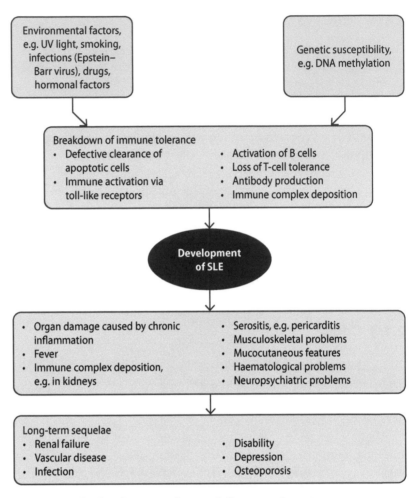

Figure 2.2. The development of systemic lupus erythematosus

2.1.4 Management

The aims of treatment are to reduce inflammation, prevent and treat disease flares and avoid long-term damage and early mortality. Symptoms may often last several months before a diagnosis is made. It is important to make a firm diagnosis and to exclude other conditions such as malignancy or infection; for example, in some cases biopsy may be needed, such as renal biopsy, to assess the degree of organ involvement and to decide on whether oral or intravenous therapy is needed. The treatment choice will depend on the disease severity, the organ involved and patient choice. SLE is a chronic condition and most patients do not achieve complete disease remission.

Non-pharmacological management

Precipitants for flares should be avoided. Sun exposure can be reduced by high sun protection factor sunscreen, clothing and hats. Patients should be encouraged to stop smoking and referred to smoking cessation services.

Physiotherapy can be helpful for tendinopathies and co-morbid conditions such as osteoarthritis. Patients who develop deformities from Jaccoud arthropathy should be referred for hand therapy.

A significant proportion of patients will suffer with low mood, anxiety and other psychological conditions, which may be due to the disease itself, e.g. neuropsychiatric involvement. Neuropsychiatric symptoms may benefit from psychological input such as cognitive behavioural therapy (CBT).

Pharmacological management

National and international guidelines advise that patient treatment is guided by severity of disease, and different regimes are suggested for mild, moderate or severe disease (see Fanouriakis *et al.*, 2019). A summary of the most common DMARDs in SLE is shown in *Table 2.1*.

Concepts of therapy in SLE

Disease activity is calculated either by BILAG or SLEDAI scores (see Isenberg *et al.*, 2005 and Ramsey-Goldman and Isenberg, 2003). The concept of treat-to-target has recently been developed in SLE, but will require further research before it is more widely adopted into clinical practice. Based on the seven clinical groups of presentation described in *Section 2.1.2*, low disease activity is considered as involvement of one to two organ systems which is controlled with low dose DMARD medication such as hydroxychloroquine; moderate disease activity may involve one or more organ systems which requires two or more DMARDs and is associated with flares; severe disease involves more than one organ system, e.g. renal,

Table 2.1. Overview of medications used to treat SLE, with mechanism of action and adverse effects

Drug		Mechanism of action	Usual level of therapy (BSR)	Screening	Adverse effects
Corticosteroids	PO/IV/IM	Works through multiple pathways including increased transcription of anti-inflammatory genes	ALL	FBC, U+Es, LFTs	Monitor for diabetes, hypertension
Hydroxychloroquine	PO	Increases lysosomal pH	ALL	Retinal screen	Retinopathy
Methotrexate	PO/SC	Dihydrofolate reductase inhibitor and increases extracellular adenosine	Moderate	Hepatitis B/C, HIV	Pneumonitis, liver toxicity, pancytopenia
Mycophenolate mofetil	PO	Inhibits T- and B-cell proliferation	Moderate	Hepatitis B/C, HIV, pregnancy test	Teratogenic, pancytopenia
Azathioprine	PO	Inhibits purine synthesis	Moderate	Hepatitis B/C, HIV	Pancytopenia
Rituximab	IV	Monoclonal antibody to CD20	Moderate/severe	Hepatitis B/C, HIV, T spot, CXR	Infusion reactions, infection (PML)
Cyclophosphamide	PO/IV	Alkylating agent	Severe	Hepatitis B/C, HIV	Teratogenic, infertility, haemorrhagic cystitis
Belimumab	IV	Monoclonal antibody against BLyS	Moderate/severe	Hepatitis B/C, HIV	Infection (PML), depression

Abbreviations: BSR, British Society for Rheumatology; PML, persistent multifocal leucoencephalopathy; CXR, chest X-ray.

but which requires prolonged therapy, often over several months or years, such as intravenous therapy, to achieve disease control. Common forms of intravenous therapy in SLE include pulsed IV cyclophosphamide or rituximab.

- **Mild disease** such as mucocutaneous and arthralgia manifestations with no organ involvement can be managed with hydroxychloroquine, although oral prednisolone may be required. Musculoskeletal manifestation can be treated with the addition of methotrexate.
- **Moderate disease** often requires higher doses of steroids and the addition of steroid-sparing agents including methotrexate, mycophenolate and azathioprine. Rituximab and belimumab can be considered in refractory cases.
- **Severe disease** includes patients with lupus nephritis and neuropsychiatric lupus, who require careful monitoring and thorough investigation. Treatment will depend on the organ involved but IV steroids will be required. Mycophenolate or cyclophosphamide are used to treat cases of lupus nephritis and refractory non-renal disease. Rituximab and belimumab can also be considered in certain cases where patients have not responded to pulsed steroids.

2.2 Sjögren's syndrome

2.2.1 Introduction

Sjögren's syndrome is a chronic autoimmune syndrome that is characterised by lymphocytic infiltration of lacrimal glands and salivary glands with subsequent symptoms of dry eyes and dry mouth. The age of onset is usually in middle age, with a population prevalence of 0.2%. Sjögren's syndrome is 20 times more common in females than in males.

2.2.2 Diagnosis

Primary Sjögren's syndrome occurs in the absence of a related condition, while secondary Sjögren's occurs in the presence of other conditions, including RA, SLE, systemic sclerosis, diabetes, chronic viral infection and autoimmune hepatitis.

Diagnosis of Sjögren's syndrome is made on clinical manifestations, antibody profile, imaging and biopsy.

Typical symptoms include:
- dryness and sicca symptoms: dry eye and dry mouth occur in most patients and require close monitoring by dentists and ophthalmologists. Patients can also present with dryness of the respiratory tract and vagina, and with cutaneous dryness causing pruritus.
- general symptoms: fatigue is common in Sjögren's. Patients also present with arthralgia, low grade fevers and widespread pain. Salivary gland swelling can occur, although infection and lymphoma must be excluded.
- organ-specific, including:
  - skin involvement with annular erythema or purpura (associated with cryoglobulinaemia)
  - respiratory involvement, most commonly with chronic obstructive or bronchiectasis picture
  - peripheral neuropathy and cranial nerve involvement can occur
  - renal involvement presents as type 1 renal tubular acidosis, membranous glomerulonephritis and membranoproliferative glomerulonephritis.

Patients with Sjögren's syndrome have a 10–44 fold increased risk of lymphoma.

Blood tests and antibody profile:
- Raised ESR and hypergammaglobulinaemia are common
- ANA positive in more than 80% of cases
- RhF positive in 50% of cases
- Extractable nuclear antigen antibodies Anti-Ro and Anti-La are associated with extraglandular features.

Imaging and biopsy:
- Schirmer's test can be used to quantify ocular dryness
- Ultrasound is often used to monitor parotid gland swelling
- Minor salivary gland biopsy showing focal lymphocytic sialadenitis is gold standard.

2.2.3 Causes

Sjögren's syndrome occurs in genetically predisposed individuals. For example, higher prevalence of Sjögren's syndrome is found in people with a family history of autoimmune conditions, including SLE and RA, who sustain environmental triggers such as infections, e.g. viruses. It is thought viral infection may lead to a dysregulated epithelium and activation of T cells and antigen-presenting cells, leading to a CD4 T-cell and B-cell response. CD4 T cells account for the majority of the lymphocytic infiltration of exocrine glands, leading to reduced function of the gland and the symptoms of dryness.

2.2.4 Management

Management is based around symptom control and prevention of complications such as infection and malignancy. This requires a comprehensive MDT approach including ophthalmologists, oral medicine specialists and rheumatologists. Sjögren's syndrome is a chronic condition and most patients do not achieve complete disease remission. National and international guidelines (Ramos-Casals *et al.*, 2020) suggest the following:

Non-pharmacological management

Non-pharmacological management plays a key role in Sjögren's syndrome. Ocular dryness can be reduced by avoiding medications which exacerbate dryness, and by the use of warm compresses, lubrication drops and punctal plugs. Oral dryness can be reduced by using sugar-free gum to stimulate salivary production, and excellent oral hygiene must be maintained.

Pharmacological management

Hydroxychloroquine can be used for skin and joint symptoms and fatigue.

A trial of pilocarpine, a muscarinic agonist, can be used to reduce ocular and oral dryness.

Occasionally DMARD therapy with methotrexate, azathioprine or mycophenolate is used for systemic complications. Cyclophosphamide, rituximab and IV Ig can be used in severe systemic complications, but this is rarely required.

2.3 Myositis

2.3.1 Introduction

Myositis per se is a very rare condition, with an estimated prevalence of 7.98 cases per million per year. Since it is very rare, there are currently no gender differences described. Age presentation varies from 30–60 years. Various distinct forms of myositis may occur, which include dermatomyositis, polymyositis and inclusion body myositis, based on clinical criteria and histological findings.

2.3.2 Diagnosis

Idiopathic inflammatory myopathies (IIM) are a group of conditions involving inflammation of muscle, associated with other systemic complications such as respiratory involvement and loss of mobility, resulting in long-term disability and impairment. Inflammatory myositis must be differentiated from other causes of proximal muscle weakness, including inherited myopathies, endocrine disorders, infections, drugs and metabolic myopathies.

The main forms of myositis include dermatomyositis, polymyositis, inclusion body myositis, juvenile dermatomyositis, cancer-associated myositis and overlap syndromes. As with other connective tissue disorders, the diagnosis can be difficult to make due to the heterogeneity of presentations. However, there are some specific syndromes presenting with typical clinical features and associated with myositis-specific antibodies.

A diagnosis of myositis should be made following exclusion of other differential diagnoses. The phenotype should then be established and complications such as interstitial lung disease and malignancy should be sought out.

The Bohan and Peter classification criteria (Bohan *et al.*, 1977) have been used for many years. More recently the EULAR/ACR criteria (Lundberg *et al.*, 2017) have been published and include key clinical, immunological and biopsy features which can be used as an aid in diagnosis.

Myositis is diagnosed based on clinical features, blood tests and biopsy results summarised below:

- **Weakness**
  - Symmetric weakness of the proximal upper extremities
  - Symmetric weakness of the proximal lower extremities
  - Neck flexors are relatively weaker than neck extensors
  - Oesophageal involvement can increase risk of aspiration and subsequent pneumonia
  - Progressive muscle weakness and inflammatory arthritis lead to reduced mobility and disability if not treated adequately.
- **Cutaneous**
  - Heliotrope rash
  - Gottron's papules
  - Gottron's sign
- **Blood tests**
  - Autoantibodies are very useful both to contribute to the diagnosis of myositis, and also to aid definition of phenotype; the most common are shown in *Table 2.2*

Table 2.2. Summary of antibodies detected in myositis

Name of antibody	Disease association
Anti-Jo1	Associated with 'Anti-synthetase syndrome', presenting with myositis, arthritis, interstitial lung disease, fever, Raynaud's and typical mechanics' hands (mechanics' hands involves thickened skin on the radial aspect and tips of the fingers)
Anti-TIF1γ	Associated with severe cutaneous disease and malignancy
Anti-NXP2	Associated with calcinosis, especially in juvenile dermatomyositis, and malignancy in adults
Anti-MDA5	Associated with interstitial lung disease and amyopathic myositis (typical skin findings but no muscle weakness)
Anti-HMGCR	Associated with statin-induced myositis
Anti-SRP	Associated with severe necrotising myositis and poor response to treatment
Anti-PM-Scl	Associated with systemic sclerosis overlap and interstitial lung disease
Anti-RNP	Associated with mixed connective tissue disease

- o CK increases with myositis and is useful in diagnosis. However, it can also be raised in many other conditions and is not always raised in idiopathic myositis. LDH, AST and ALT can also be raised.
- **Biopsy**
  - o In dermatomyositis the biopsy will show perivascular infiltrates with CD4+, macrophages and occasional B cells, whereas in polymyositis the biopsy will show more CD8 T cells within the muscle fascicles. Rimmed vacuoles are typical for inclusion body myositis.
- **MRI**
  - o MRI is sensitive for muscle inflammation and is used to identify active myositis and site for biopsy
  - o Electromyography (EMG) is used to exclude neurological disorders and assess severity of disease.
- **Pulmonary investigations**
  - o Lung involvement is a cause of mortality in up to 80% of cases with inflammatory myositis. The most common pattern is non-specific interstitial pneumonia (NSIP), characterised by inflammatory infiltrate and ground glass changes in the lower zones. Patients can present with progressive breathlessness, and ultimately lung fibrosis can lead to pulmonary arterial hypertension and right heart failure.
- **Malignancy**
  - o Myositis is associated with increased risk of malignancy. Therefore, all patients should have thorough screening for malignancy. The most common cancers associated with myositis are lung, ovary, non-Hodgkin lymphoma, gastrointestinal (GI) and breast.

Myositis is rare, but the more common manifestations of the IIM diseases are summarised below.

Dermatomyositis

Dermatomyositis presents with pathognomonic rashes which can precede muscle involvement. Gottron's papules are raised red lesions on the dorsal aspect of metacarpophalangeal (MCP) and interphalangeal joints, whilst Gottron's sign are macules over the extensor surfaces of other joints. Photosensitive erythematous rash can occur over the upper back (shawl sign), anterior chest (V sign) and over the hips (holster sign). Patients with dermatomyositis will often suffer from Raynaud's and have nailfold telangiectasia and 'ragged cuticles'.

Polymyositis

Polymyositis is a painless slowly progressive muscle weakness which affects the proximal muscle groups of the arms and the legs. Patients may present with difficulty standing from a chair, climbing stairs and reaching for objects in cupboards. Oesophageal muscles can also be affected and present as dysphagia and gastro-oesophageal reflux. More rarely, cardiac muscle can be involved, leading to conduction abnormalities and arrhythmia. Diagnosis is made based on clinical features, raised muscle CK levels, evidence of polyphasic features on nerve conduction and muscle biopsy.

2.3.3 Causes

The cause and pathogenesis of idiopathic myositis is not completely understood. GWAS have identified human leucocyte antigen genes and genes for antibody profiles which are associated with myositis. Certain drugs, such as statins, are known triggers of myositis but seem to be separate entities with different biopsy findings and response to treatment. Viral infections such as HIV, influenza and Coxsackie virus have also been implicated in triggering myositis, but their exact role is unclear.

The CD4 cell-rich infiltrate found on biopsies implies a key role for T cells and the adaptive immune system. B cells are less prevalent in tissue; however, the key role of autoantibodies suggests some involvement of the humoral response. There is also evidence of an innate response with activation of TLRs and expression of tumour necrosis factor alpha (TNF-α) and IL-1. Lastly, it has also been proposed that endoplasmic reticulum stress response may lead to non-immune muscle fibre destruction.

2.3.4 Management

Management decisions in myositis will depend on clinical phenotype, severity of disease and presence of complications. Myositis is a chronic condition and most patients do not achieve complete disease remission.

Non-pharmacological management

Physiotherapy and exercise are crucial in the recovery from myositis and all patients should have access to specialist physiotherapy services.

Pharmacological management

The mainstay of treatment is glucocorticoids, which treat musculo-skeletal, cutaneous and respiratory complications. If disease is severe then IV methylprednisolone is given, which can act more rapidly than oral glucocorticoids, followed by weaning high dose prednisolone which needs to be closely monitored and slowly weaned.

DMARDs are usually initiated to allow the weaning of steroids, which have significant morbidity burden. There is only a small evidence base for immunosuppressive therapy in myositis, with most evidence coming from case series or small trials. The most commonly used DMARDs in the UK are azathioprine and methotrexate, but ciclosporin, tacrolimus and mycophenolate are also used.

In cases of severe disease with lung involvement, dysphagia and severe weakness, cyclophosphamide IV is used. IV Ig can also be used in those with dysphagia and severe skin disease, but patients tend to relapse once therapy is stopped and so treatment is limited by cost and the long-term effects of IV Ig therapy.

Reponses to biological therapy such as anti-TNF and anti-IL1 have been disappointing. However, rituximab has now been licensed for use in active myositis which has failed conventional therapy.

2.4 Systemic sclerosis

2.4.1 Introduction

The incidence of scleroderma is estimated at 27 new cases per million population per year. There is a preponderance for females (3:1) and it usually presents between 30 and 50 years of age. It may be preceded by symptoms of Raynaud's phenomenon for many years.

2.4.2 Diagnosis

Systemic sclerosis is a chronic autoimmune condition which affects the skin and internal organs. Limited systemic sclerosis involves skin distal to the elbows and knees, with a slower progression of skin thickening and later onset of complications which include pulmonary hypertension and GI dysmotility. It is associated with anti-centromere antibodies. Diffuse systemic sclerosis involves skin proximal to the elbows and knees and generally has a faster onset of skin thickening and internal organ involvement including lung fibrosis, renal crisis and myocardial involvement. Systemic sclerosis can overlap with conditions such as myositis and SLE.

As with other conditions in this chapter there are no diagnostic criteria, but classification criteria can be used to identify patients with distinct symptoms. The 2013 ACR/EULAR criteria are shown in *Table 2.3*.

Systemic sclerosis is caused by a triad of vasculopathy, fibrosis and autoimmune activation, and clinical presentations and treatment reflect this. Early diagnosis is key to prevent damage and complications. Clinical features are associated with multisystem involvement and can be categorised with respect to the groupings below:

Table 2.3. 2013 ACR/EULAR criteria for systemic sclerosis

Items	Sub-items	Score
Skin thickening of the fingers of both hands extending proximal to the MCP joints		9
Skin thickening of fingers	Puffy fingers	2
Only count highest score	Whole finger, distal to MCP joint	4
Fingertip lesions	Digital tip ulcers	2
Only count highest score	Pitting scars	3
Telangiectasia		2
Abnormal nailfold capillaries		2
Pulmonary arterial hypertension and/or interstitial lung disease		2
Raynaud's		3
Antibodies (anti-centromere, anti-ScL 70, anti-RNA polymerase III)		3
Patients with a score of ≥9 have definite systemic sclerosis		

Vascular changes

Raynaud's is usually the first symptom and should be investigated with autoimmune profile and nailfold capillaroscopy, which can be abnormal even in early disease.

Digital ulcers can occur as a result of severe Raynaud's and ischaemia which can be very difficult to treat. They are prone to infection and heal slowly due to the poor blood supply.

Pulmonary arterial hypertension is a leading cause of mortality but is difficult to diagnose and is asymptomatic in the early stages. Therefore, regular screening with brain natriuretic peptide (BNP), echocardiogram to estimate pulmonary artery pressures and lung function tests for diffuse capacity of the lungs for carbon monoxide (DLCO) are recommended. However, the gold standard for diagnosis is right heart catheterisation which should be performed in a specialist centre. Anti-centromere antibodies are associated with the development of pulmonary arterial hypertension.

Fibrosis and autoimmune activation

Systemic sclerosis can affect the whole GI tract. The most common presentation is gastro-oesophageal reflux due to altered oesophageal motility. This should be investigated with endoscopy and oesophageal motility studies and patients should be screened for Barrett's oesophagus. Patients have a higher incidence of gastric antral vascular ectasia, which presents with anaemia due to dilated blood vessels in the antrum of the stomach. Altered small bowel motility can result in small bowel bacterial overgrowth and malabsorption symptoms. Anorectal scleroderma can also occur and require nerve stimulator therapy.

Interstitial lung fibrosis is a key predictor of morbidity and mortality. HRCT is the gold standard investigation to identify this and NSIP is the most common pattern. Lung function tests including DLCO can also be used to screen and to determine treatment choices. Lung fibrosis is associated with anti-Scl 70/anti-topoisomerase I antibody positivity.

Cardiac involvement includes cardiac fibrosis, pericarditis and arrhythmia. Again, thorough examination and investigation is required to make a diagnosis as symptoms are often non-specific and mild. Pericarditis in particular is associated with renal crisis and can lead to tamponade.

Scleroderma renal crisis presents as malignant hypertension with headaches, visual changes, seizures and acute pulmonary oedema with pericardial effusion, microangiopathic haemolytic anaemia and renal failure. There is evidence it can be triggered by high dose steroids so they should be used cautiously in these patients, especially in those who are positive for anti-RNA polymerase III, which is associated with risk of renal crisis.

2.4.3 Causes

The cause of systemic sclerosis is not understood. There is familial clustering and so some genetic component. It is then thought a triggering event occurs, which is amplified either by genetic or immunological predisposition followed by progression of disease. Some agents which cause a scleroderma-like presentation, such as the chemotherapy agent taxane, vinyl chloride and solvents, have been implicated as the environmental trigger. Infectious agents may also play a part. Overall, systemic sclerosis pathology is due to vasculopathy, immune activation and fibrosis. These three pathologies are important in understanding the clinical presentation and treatment of disease.

2.4.4 Management

International guidelines on the treatment of systemic sclerosis have been published (van den Hoogen *et al.*, 2013). This highlights the importance of early diagnosis and treatment to aim to prevent disease progression. Once diagnosed, patients are managed in a specialist centre and treatment is aimed at the organ involved. Scleroderma is a chronic condition and most patients do not achieve complete disease remission.

Non-pharmacological management

Patients with Raynaud's should be advised to keep hands and central body warm. Patients with ulcers need to closely monitor them for signs of infection. Itch can be a major issue and patients should have access to moisturisers and antihistamines. Telangiectasia can sometimes be treated with laser.

Pharmacological management

First-line pharmacological treatment for Raynaud's are calcium channel blockers and angiotensin 2 blockers. Selective serotonin reuptake inhibitors, alpha blockers and phosphodiesterase type 5 inhibitors are also used. IV iloprost can be used in refractory and severe cases. Digital sympathectomy can also be used in severe cases.

Diffuse skin fibrosis can be treated with methotrexate, mycophenolate or cyclophosphamide.

Most patients will suffer with reflux, which can be treated with PPIs, histamine H2 receptor antagonists or, sometimes, prokinetic dopamine antagonists. Symptomatic agents such as loperamide can be useful in chronic diarrhoea. Antibiotic courses are sometimes required in bacterial overgrowth.

Patients at risk of renal disease should have their blood pressure monitored regularly. Renal crisis is treated with angiotensin-converting enzyme inhibitor and all patients should be monitored closely in a high dependency unit setting.

All patients should be evaluated for pulmonary arterial hypertension (PAH) and lung fibrosis.

PAH needs to be diagnosed early and patients with PAH should be reviewed by a specialist centre.

Lung fibrosis can be treated with cyclophosphamide followed by azathioprine or mycophenolate.

Autologous haemopoietic stem cell transplant can be considered in patients with severe diffuse cutaneous systemic sclerosis who do not have severe internal organ disease that would mean the risks are too high.

2.5 Cases

The following case histories are real-life examples demonstrating diagnosis and decision-making processes.

Case history 2.1

A 26-year-old man comes to clinic with a history of the tips of his fingers turning white, blue and then red, triggered by cold, in a symmetrical distribution. He is concerned because, although he has had this since being a teenager, it has been getting worse over the last 6 months. He has no other medical history.

He has no other symptoms on systems review. His general practitioner (GP) has requested initial bloods which show:
- ANA negative
- RhF negative, anti-CCP negative
- Complement normal
- Hepatitis B, C and HIV negative

What is the differential diagnosis of Raynaud's syndrome?

Raynaud's may be primary (idiopathic) or secondary to another condition. Secondary causes include those in *Table 2.4*.

What investigation would be most helpful to confirm your diagnosis?

- Anti-DsDNA
- Cryoglobulins
- Chest X-ray (CXR)
- Nailfold capillaroscopy
- Ultrasound (US) Doppler arms

The history is suggestive of primary Raynaud's in an otherwise well man with long-standing symptoms of symmetrical Raynaud's and no ulceration. It is unlikely to be related to a connective tissue disorder with a negative ANA and normal nailfold capillaroscopy, so nailfold capillaroscopy would be the most useful test.

He is keen to be treated for his Raynaud's as it is now bothering him, especially in the winter. His GP has already advised him to avoid the cold, ensure good body heating, buy heated gloves and stop smoking.

What intervention would you suggest?

- Bisoprolol
- Clopidogrel
- Digital sympathectomy
- IV iloprost
- Nifedipine

There is limited evidence for all medications in Raynaud's. However, the National Institute for Health and Care Excellence (NICE) suggests a trial of calcium antagonists, e.g. nifedipine or amlodipine, in those individuals where lifestyle measures are unsuccessful. Intravenous iloprost and, in severe cases, digital sympathectomy, can be used for very severe Raynaud's or digital ulceration. Clopidogrel is not recommended for treatment of Raynaud's. Beta blockers such as bisoprolol can make Raynaud's worse.

Table 2.4. Causes of Raynaud's syndrome

Connective tissue diseases	Increased viscosity	Vascular	Endocrine	Drugs	Environmental
Scleroderma	Polycythaemia	Occlusive/ atherosclerosis	Carcinoid syndrome	Beta blocker	Smoking
SLE	Cryoglobulin-aemia	Buerger's disease	Phaeochro-mocytoma	Ergot derivatives	Vibration white finger
Dermatomyositis	MGUS	Takayasu's arteritis	Diabetes mellitus	Chemotherapy	
Sjögren's syndrome	Cold agglutinins	Giant cell arteritis			
Rheumatoid arthritis					

Abbreviation: MGUS, multiple myeloma undetermined significance.

Case history 2.2

A 60-year-old lady comes to rheumatology clinic. 30 years ago she was diagnosed with SLE based on a butterfly rash, myositis and positive serology, being ANA, anti-dsDNA and anti-Ro positive. She was started on hydroxychloroquine at this time but has been taking it intermittently for the last 10 years as her symptoms have not been troubling her.

Over the last 2 months she has developed pain and stiffness in the small joints of her hands and in her shoulders. On examination she has an ongoing mild malar rash and florid synovitis of her MCP and proximal interphalangeal (PIP) joints.

What is the next test you would do?

- Aspiration of MCP joints
- Chest X-ray (CXR)
- MRI hands
- RhF and anti-CCP antibodies
- Skin biopsy malar rash

The next test would be RhF and anti-CCP antibodies to fully elucidate her immunological profile. MRI hands would not add to your clinical information as you already know she has synovitis from examination.

RhF and anti-CCP come back strongly positive, and so with evidence of active synovitis and the clear history of SLE a diagnosis of 'rhupus' (a combination of RA and SLE features in the same patient), or RA and SLE overlap syndrome, is made.

She is given oral prednisolone weaning regime and started on methotrexate. She is unable to tolerate methotrexate and has ongoing active disease so rituximab treatment is started. Rituximab is licensed for the treatment of RA and is used particularly in those who are seropositive. It is also used in the treatment of SLE and so will have beneficial effects for both her SLE and rheumatoid manifestations.

She has a good clinical response to this but begins to get recurrent chest infections.

What is the next course of action?

- Bone marrow biopsy
- Check immunoglobulin levels
- Positron emission tomography (PET) scan
- Stop biologic as it is now contraindicated
- Switch her to adalimumab

Rituximab is a monoclonal antibody against CD20, which is expressed on immature B cells. Rituximab therapy leads to the depletion of B cells and in turn reduction in immunoglobulin production by plasma cells. B-cell deficiency is known to predispose to recurrent chest infections and so it would be appropriate to measure immunoglobulin levels in this patient. In practice immunoglobulin levels should be checked prior to each rituximab course.

Case history 2.3

A 28-year-old lady known to the rheumatology team is admitted via the ED with absence episodes. She is known to have SLE based on photosensitive rash, arthralgia and positive ANA and anti-dsDNA.

Which other antibody would you like to test for?

- Anti-Jo 1
- Anti-ribosomal antibodies
- Anti-RNP
- Anti-Ro
- Anti-Sm

Anti-ribosomal antibodies are associated with cerebral lupus.

You review her on the acute medical unit. She has been having absence episodes 6–8 times a day with significant post ictal periods. On further questioning she tells you about both auditory and visual hallucinations consisting of loud noises, shadows and feelings of dissociation. The medical team have excluded infection and the neurological team have initiated anti-epileptic medication which seems to be helping.

Which immunosuppressant would you prescribe once the diagnosis of cerebral lupus is confirmed?

- Azathioprine
- Belimumab
- Cyclophosphamide
- Methotrexate
- Oral steroids

This lady has a severe flare of neuropsychiatric SLE and so the most appropriate immunosuppressant would be IV cyclophosphamide (British Society for Rheumatology (BSR) guidelines). This lady is of child-bearing age and so she will need to be counselled regarding the risks of infertility and the need to use adequate contraception, as cyclophosphamide is teratogenic. Cyclophosphamide will be given with IV methylprednisolone and then oral steroids. Methotrexate and azathioprine would not be appropriate as they take too long to be efficacious, although azathioprine may be considered as maintenance therapy. Belimumab is not currently offered for renal or neuropsychiatric SLE but studies are currently underway to test its efficacy in this setting.

The patient significantly improves and you see her in clinic 5 years later. She has remained well during this time and now wishes to discuss the possibility of trying for a baby (she is aware of the risks of infertility from her previous treatment). You review her previous immunology which is as follows:
- ANA positive
- Anti-dsDNA positive
- Anti-Ro and -La positive

- Ribosomal antibody positive
- Negative anti-Sm antibody
- Negative antiphospholipid screen

Which of these complications of pregnancy is most likely, given the fact she is anti-Ro/-La positive?

- Congenital heart block
- Hypertension
- Intrauterine growth restriction
- Neonatal skin rash
- Post-partum haemorrhage

A rash similar to subacute cutaneous lupus, with erythema and central clearing, a few weeks after birth will occur in about 5% of babies born to anti-Ro positive mothers. This will resolve in the majority of cases. Congenital heart block occurs in 1–2% babies and usually does not resolve, with babies requiring a pacemaker in the first years of life. Patients with SLE are at increased risk of pre-eclampsia and of delivering babies prematurely or with intrauterine growth restriction. For this reason patients with SLE are closely monitored in pregnancy, and those who are Ro/La positive will have regular fetal heart monitoring during pregnancy.

Case history 2.4

A 71-year-old woman with Sjögren's syndrome comes for review. She has long-standing sicca symptoms and is anti-Ro and -La positive. She takes hydroxychloroquine daily along with her eye drops. She has not been feeling well recently, although she cannot put her finger on it.

Which of the below is a known complication of Sjögren's?

- B12 deficiency anaemia (pernicious anaemia)
- Diabetes mellitus
- Flu
- Lymphoma
- TB

Patients with Sjögren's syndrome have increased risk of developing lymphoma and so should be carefully evaluated at each visit for this. The most common lymphomas are diffuse large B-cell lymphoma and mucosa-associated lymphoid tissue (MALT) lymphomas. Any patient presenting with lymph gland swelling or parotid swelling should undergo imaging ± biopsy.

Following an excision biopsy, CT PET and bone marrow biopsy, a diagnosis of MALT lymphoma was made and she was treated with radiotherapy.

She remains stable on review in clinic for a number of years. However, during a busy clinic, although she remains well she mentions a new rash on her lower legs.

What is the next test you would request to confirm your suspicions?

- ANCA
- Arterial Doppler
- Cryoglobulins
- Hepatitis screen
- Venous Doppler

Systemic sclerosis can be associated with cryoglobulinaemic vasculitis. A skin biopsy would also be useful to help make the diagnosis. Cryoglobulinaemia can be divided into:
- Type 1 monoclonal antibody, typically associated with lymphoproliferative disorders such as MGUS or multiple myeloma
- 'Mixed cryoglobulinaemia: type 2 (monoclonal IgM with polyclonal IgG) and type 3 (polyclonal IgM plus polyclonal IgG or IgA), typically associated with infections such as hepatitis C and HIV and autoimmune conditions such as Sjögren's syndrome, RA and SLE.

Cryoglobulin levels and skin biopsy confirm your diagnosis. You start her on azathioprine in addition to her hydroxychloroquine.

Case history 2.5

A 32-year-old female is admitted following a 6-month history of proximal muscle weakness and generalised fatigue. Her muscles are tender to touch and she has become housebound in the last 3 months. She has no symptoms of dysphagia but she has noticed some shortness of breath. On examination she has proximal muscle weakness and thickening and cracking of the skin on the sides of her fingers. Initial tests reveal CK is 10 000 and MRI thigh and EMG are consistent with inflammatory myopathy. Electrocardiogram (ECG) and troponin are normal.

Which antibody is classically associated with this condition?

- Anti-centromere
- Anti-Jo1
- Anti-Sm
- Anti-SRP
- Anti-TIF1γ

Anti-synthetase syndrome is classically associated with anti-Jo1 antibodies. The syndrome typically presents with inflammatory myositis, interstitial lung disease, 'mechanics' hands' and inflammatory arthritis. Although patients with anti-synthetase syndrome are still at risk of cancer, the risk is lower than with other forms of inflammatory myositis. Anti-synthetase syndrome is most common in females, and although it typically presents around the age of 50, it can occur in younger and older patients.

You request an HRCT scan to investigate her breathlessness further. What pattern would you typically see?

- Usual interstitial pneumonia
- NSIP
- Chronic hypersensitivity pneumonitis
- Lymphadenopathy
- Apical fibrosis

Her CT shows NSIP which is typically seen in myositis, although other patterns of fibrosis such as organising pneumonia can be present. Lung function tests would show a restrictive pattern with a reduced carbon monoxide transfer factor. Bronchoalveolar lavage may be used to assess disease activity and exclude other causes of ILD.

How would you treat her initially?

- IV methylprednisolone followed by oral prednisolone
- Methotrexate
- Azathioprine
- Plasma exchange
- Ciclosporin

This lady needs to have high dose steroids, which are the mainstay of treatment, to get her disease under control. She is given IV methylprednisolone followed by high dose oral prednisolone on a slow weaning regime. She significantly improves with this. Her long-term immunosuppression is discussed with the respiratory team and it is decided to start methotrexate.

She recovers from this flare and is seen in clinic 2 years later stable on methotrexate. She is keen to consider pregnancy now.

What is the most appropriate plan for her medication?

- Switch to azathioprine
- Continue methotrexate with current folic acid dose
- Continue methotrexate but increase the folic acid dose
- Stop DMARDs and give steroids instead
- Switch to leflunomide

Methotrexate and leflunomide are both contraindicated in pregnancy, and leflunomide is not usually used in myositis. Azathioprine would be a reasonable option to switch to and is safe in pregnancy and breastfeeding.

See BSR guidelines on DMARDs/biologics in pregnancy (Flint *et al.*, 2016).

Three years later the patient re-presents with increasing proximal muscle weakness, joint synovitis and increasing shortness of breath. She has been taking her azathioprine as prescribed. She is very concerned as she wishes to try for another baby in the near future.

What treatment would you consider now?

- Leflunomide
- Naproxen
- Rituximab
- Belimumab
- Cyclophosphamide

Rituximab and cyclophosphamide could be used to control her relapse. However, rituximab would be the best option in this case. Cyclophosphamide is known to be highly teratogenic and can cause infertility. Patients should not become pregnant until at least 6 months after receiving cyclophosphamide. Rituximab also should not be used in pregnancy and it is recommended by BSR that it should be stopped at least 6 months prior to conception. However, it does not cause infertility, and unintentional first trimester exposure is unlikely to be harmful.

Rituximab can be used in patients who have failed (including contraindications or severe adverse effects) with conventional treatment including corticosteroids and at least two immunosuppressive steroid-sparing drugs. As this lady has a contraindication to methotrexate and has failed azathioprine, she is eligible for treatment.

Case history 2.6

A 38-year-old lady comes to clinic. She gives a history of developing dry itchy skin about 2 years previously which her GP treated with creams. She then developed Raynaud's and intermittent paraesthesia in the tips of her fingers. Over the last couple of months, she has noticed some tightening of the skin on her neck and chest which has prompted her referral to you. On systems review she reveals she has been suffering from shortness of breath on walking her dog in the mornings which she had not noticed previously. She has also had an increase in GI reflux symptoms. On examination you find skin thickening in both hands and on her chest and neck.

Which antibody are you most interested in seeing the result of?

- Anti-dsDNA
- Anti-U1RNP
- Anti-centromere
- Anti-ScL 70
- RhF

This lady fulfils the 2013 ACR/EULAR criteria for systemic sclerosis and she has thickening of the skin proximal to her elbows so has diffuse cutaneous systemic sclerosis. She has some progressive shortness of breath which may be a symptom of ILD, and anti-ScL 70 is associated with this. Anti-centromere antibody is associated with limited cutaneous systemic sclerosis. Anti-dsDNA is associated with SLE and anti-U1RNP is associated with mixed connective tissue disease.

She comes back as ANA and anti-ScL 70 antibody positive.

What investigations would you like to request?

The patient has diffuse cutaneous systemic sclerosis and is at risk of rapid progression and complications. Therefore, early recognition of complications is important. She needs renal function and blood pressure monitored. She needs Nt-proBNP, troponin, ECG and echocardiogram to look for cardiac involvement. The echocardiogram will be important to screen for PAH along with lung function tests for DLCO. Lung function test and HRCT should be requested to screen for lung fibrosis. She needs an upper GI endoscopy ± manometry.

Her HRCT shows some mild interstitial lung disease but her lung function tests are normal. Otherwise, her investigations are normal.

You continue to follow her up in clinic and are giving her nifedipine for her troublesome Raynaud's symptoms, with omeprazole and ranitidine for her gastro-oesophageal reflux. About 4 months later she presents with a deep ulcer on her index finger which looks partly necrotic and is extremely painful.

What treatment would you give her now?
- Arrange for amputation
- Aspirin
- Flucloxacillin
- Increase nifedipine dose
- Iloprost infusion

She is admitted to the day unit for urgent iloprost infusions. Nifedipine can be used in Raynaud's but will not improve active ulceration.

At next review she mentions that her respiratory symptoms are worsening and she is becoming progressively more short of breath. Her lung function tests have worsened and so you decide to start her on mycophenolate.

One month later you are called by the cardiology registrar. She has been admitted overnight with chest pain and a large pericardial effusion which required pericardiocentesis. CT chest, which has been performed, shows marked interstitial lung disease. On review her skin has also worsened and she has developed another digital ulcer.

What treatment would you give now?
- Colchicine
- Cyclophosphamide
- Increase mycophenolate
- Methotrexate
- Pirfenidone

She has had an overall deterioration, including progression of her lung fibrosis, despite mycophenolate. Cyclophosphamide would be appropriate in this setting and discussion with a specialist centre regarding ongoing treatment would be needed. Methotrexate can be used for early skin involvement but not in severe systemic disease. Colchicine would not be used. Pirfenidone is an antifibrotic used in idiopathic pulmonary fibrosis.

2.6 References

Aringer, M., Costenbader, K., Daikh, D. *et al.* (2019) 2019 European League Against Rheumatism/American College of Rheumatology classification criteria for systemic lupus erythematosus. *Ann Rheum Dis.*, **78**: 1151–1159.

Bohan, A., Peter, J.B., Bowman, R.L. *et al.* (1977) Computer-assisted analysis of 153 patients with polymyositis and dermatomyositis. *Medicine (Baltimore)*, **56(4)**: 255–286.

Fanouriakis, A., Kostopoulou, M., Alunno, A. *et al.* (2019) 2019 update of the EULAR recommendations for the management of systemic lupus erythematosus. *Ann Rheum Dis.*, **78**: 736–745.

Flint, J., Panchal, S., Hurrell, A. *et al.* (2016) BSR and BHPR guideline on prescribing drugs in pregnancy and breastfeeding—Part I: standard and biologic disease modifying anti-rheumatic drugs and corticosteroids. *Rheumatology*, **55**: 1693–1697.

Hochberg, M.C. (1997) Updating the American College of Rheumatology revised criteria for the classification of systemic lupus erythematosus. *Arthritis Rheum.*, **40(9)**: 1725.

Isenberg, D.A., Rahman, A., Allen, E. *et al.* (2005) BILAG 2004. Development and initial validation of an updated version of the British Isles Lupus Assessment Group's disease activity index for patients with systemic lupus erythematosus. *Rheumatology (Oxford)*, **44(7)**: 902–906.

Lundberg, I.E., Tjärnlund, A., Bottai, M. *et al.* (2017) EULAR/ACR classification criteria for adult and juvenile idiopathic inflammatory myopathies and their major subgroups. *Ann Rheum Dis.*, **76(12)**: 1955–1964.

Mayes, M.D. (1998) Classification and epidemiology of scleroderma. *Semin Cutan Med Surg.*, **17(1)**: 22–26.

Meyer, A., Meyer, N., Schaeffer, M. *et al.* (2015) Incidence and prevalence of inflammatory myopathies: a systematic review. *Rheumatology (Oxford)*, **54**: 50–63.

Petri, M., Orbai, A-M., Alarcón, G.S. *et al.* (2012) Derivation and validation of the Systemic Lupus International Collaborating Clinics classification criteria for systemic lupus erythematosus. *Arthritis Rheum.*, **64(8)**: 2677–2686.

Ramsey-Goldman, R. and Isenberg, D.A. (2003) Systemic lupus erythematosus measures: British Isles Lupus Assessment Group (BILAG), European Consensus Lupus Activity Measurement (ECLAM), Systemic Lupus Activity Measure (SLAM), Systemic Lupus Erythematosus Disease Activity Measure (SLEDAI), and Systemic Lupus International Collaborating Clinics/American College of Rheumatology-Damage Index (SLICC/ACR-DI; SDI). *Arthritis Care & Research*, **49**: S225–S233.

Ramos-Casals, M., Brito-Zerón, P., Bombardieri, S. *et al.* (2020) EULAR recommendations for the management of Sjögren's syndrome with topical and systemic therapies. *Ann Rheum Dis.*, **79(1):** 3–18.

van den Hoogen, F., Khanna, D., Fransen, J. *et al.* (2013) Classification criteria for systemic sclerosis: an ACR-EULAR collaborative initiative. *Arthritis Rheum.*, **65(11):** 2737–2747.

NICE, BSR guidelines and useful websites

NICE guidelines for the management of SLE, Raynaud's, scleroderma and myositis
https://cks.nice.org.uk/raynauds-phenomenon#!scenario

www.england.nhs.uk/wp-content/uploads/2018/07/Rituximab-for-the-treatment-of-dermatomyositis-and-polymyositis-adults.pdf

BSR guidelines

https://academic.oup.com/rheumatology/article/55/10/1906/2196591
https://academic.oup.com/rheumatology/article/57/1/e1/4318863

CHAPTER 3

Crystal arthropathies

In this chapter we discuss the diagnosis, pathophysiology and management of gout and calcium pyrophosphate deposition disease (CPPD). Crystal arthropathies include the most common inflammatory arthropathies worldwide. The real-life cases will provide an insight into diagnostic issues and long-term management. We also discuss new therapies available for resistant cases and acute attacks of gout, including biologic and enzymatic treatments.

3.1 Gout

3.1.1 Introduction

Gout is the most prevalent inflammatory arthropathy in populations worldwide. Gout has a prevalence of up to 2.5% in Europe (Bardin *et al.*, 2016), 3.9 % in the USA (Zhu *et al.*, 2011) and more than 6% in some Asia-Pacific countries (Kuo *et al.*, 2015a). Gout is predominantly a condition affecting men, with a ratio of approximately 4.3:1 in the UK. Gout prevalence varies in different populations and is reported at a higher prevalence in North America and among indigenous populations such as Maori, Aboriginals and Inuit. In recent times there has been an increase in women. The age of onset is typically between 30 and 50 years. Gout is rare below the age of 20 and tends to plateau around the age of 80.

Gout is a condition characterised by acute episodes of inflammation, which should be controlled as rapidly as possible to achieve optimal control. It is important to make a diagnosis of gout, since there are modifiable risk factors and treatments which can be administered to achieve optimal control.

3.1.2 Diagnosis

Gout is often misdiagnosed without adequate clinical, biochemical and/or radiological work-up, therefore correct diagnosis and management is key. In recent years, several evidence-based recommendations have been made for the diagnosis and treatment of gout, which will be referred to in this chapter (Richette *et al.*, 2020; Hui *et al.*, 2017).

Monosodium urate (MSU) crystals are normally detected under polarised light microscopy in synovial fluid aspirated from symptomatic and asymptomatic joints. MSU crystals are rod- or needle-shaped and show negative birefringence under polarised light. The most commonly affected joint in gout is the first metatarsophalangeal (MTP) joint. Since crystals can also be isolated during an asymptomatic inter-critical period, or between joint flares, a diagnosis of gout can also be made in between joint flares.

Plain radiographs are often performed at the time of presentation and may be normal. Other changes which can be observed include non-specific soft tissue swelling and subcortical cysts. In advanced disease, punched-out bone erosions are often observed.

3.1.3 Causes

Gout is due to the development of prolonged hyperuricaemia. A rise in systemic uric acid leads to the formation of MSU crystals which can then accumulate in joints and other tissues, e.g. underneath the skin, to form gouty tophi. Gout is caused by several factors leading to the accumulation of MSU crystals in the tissues and joints and represents a response by the host in reaction to MSU crystals. The gold standard remains the detection of MSU crystals in fluid or tophus aspirates, as it has 100% specificity. Uric acid is formed from the degradation of purine and is mainly formed in the liver. Most uric acid is excreted by the kidney and a smaller proportion is secreted into the intestine.

Once MSU crystals form and deposit in the joint, the host response triggers the clinical syndrome of gout (see *Figure 3.1*).

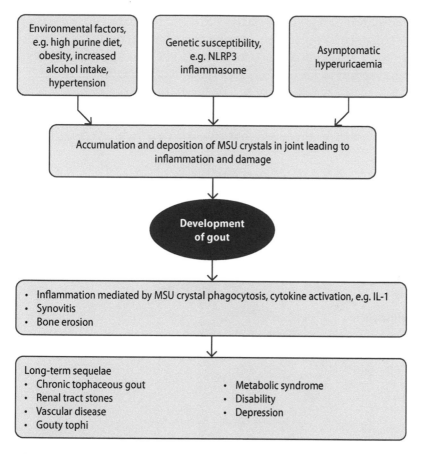

Figure 3.1. The development of gout

Acute gout occurs due to the infiltration and phagocytosis by polymorphonuclear lymphocytes of new crystals formed in the joint. Crystals are coated with IgG, which reacts with Fc receptors on polymorphonuclear cells that phagocytose the crystals. Within the cell, MSU crystals are stripped of their protein coats and then release a number of inflammatory mediators.

Most cases of gout are caused by the underexcretion of uric acid. The serum levels of urate correlate directly with the risk of disease. However, gout can occur in people with normal plasma urate levels and many people with asymptomatic hyperuricaemia do not develop gout. Other rarer but important causes of gout include inherited enzyme defects (hypoxanthine-guanine phosphoribosyltransferase (HGPRT) deficiency, or overactivity of phosphoribosyl pyrophosphate (PRPP) synthetase). Acute gout can be triggered by high alcohol intake, dehydration, purine-rich foods, drugs (e.g. loop diuretics), surgery, trauma and infection. Alcohol raises serum lactate levels, which block renal excretion of urate.

The long-term burden of disease in gout can be reduced by preventing the deposition of MSU crystals. At the earliest stages, uric acid levels may be high in the blood, but subjects may not have any clinical

Table 3.1. Summary of the causes of hyperuricaemia

Causes of hyperuricaemia	Conditions
Overproduction Increased uric acid production or increased purine synthesis Conditions linked to purine overproduction	Congenital enzyme defects
	Hypoxanthine-guanine phosphoribosyltransferase (HGPRT) deficiency
	Complete (Lesch–Nyhan syndrome), incomplete
	PRPP synthetase overactivity
	Haemolytic conditions
	Lymphoproliferative and myeloproliferative conditions
	Neoplasms
	Obesity
Undersecretion Reduced renal clearance of uric acid	Primary idiopathic uric acid undersecretion
	Secondary uric acid undersecretion due to: • chronic renal failure • congestive heart failure • dehydration • hypothyroidism • hyperparathyroidism • hypertension • ischaemic heart disease
Drugs	Ciclosporin
	Diuretics, especially loop diuretics
	Ethanol
	Ethambutol
	Levodopa
	Low-dose salicylate
	Pyrazinamide

features of gout. When MSU crystals deposit in joints and other tissue, overtly clinical features develop such as a gout flare, chronic gouty arthritis and the development of tophi. Often acute gout flares may be separated by periods of asymptomatic disease. The aims of therapy are to prevent acute attacks and prevent further deposition of MSU crystals.

Uric acid exists as sodium urate at physiological pH. An elevated level of MSU can be caused by overproduction or decreased renal clearance of urate (*Table 3.1*).

3.1.4 Management

The management of gout can be divided into acute and chronic phases (based on NICE guidelines – https://cks.nice.org.uk/gout). Acute attacks should be treated as early as possible, to ease symptoms and to prevent the development of long-term sequelae.

Non-pharmacological management

Acute gout

The patient should be advised to rest and elevate the limb. Any trauma should be avoided to the affected joint. As much as possible, the joint should be kept exposed and placed in a cool environment. Consider the use of an ice-pack or a bed-cage.

In order to prevent future attacks, lifestyle issues should be discussed such as weight loss, exercise, a healthy low purine diet, reduction of alcohol consumption and maintaining fluid intake with water-based beverages.

Chronic gout

- Lifestyle advice – since many attacks of gout can be precipitated by episodes such as dehydration, heavy alcohol intake or intercurrent illness, advice on lifestyle changes should be given to prevent further episodes; for example, maintaining adequate hydration, reducing high alcohol intake and treating risk factors such as hypertension. Adequate exercise, controlling weight and a low purine diet are all part of lifestyle recommendations that should be given to people with recurrent episodes of gout.

Pharmacological management

The pharmacological agents used for the management of acute and chronic gout are summarised in *Table 3.2*. Principles of management for acute gout are to suppress acute pain and inflammation. For chronic gout, medications for ULT are recommended.

Urate-lowering therapy (ULT) is recommended in the management of chronic gout to prevent long-term damage (e.g. joint erosions and renal tract stones) and to prevent flares. The aim of ULT is to reduce serum uric acid concentration to <300 micromol/L.

Acute gout

Provided there are no contraindications, an NSAID at a maximum dose as early as possible is recommended, with continuation at the maximum daily dose until 1–2 days after the attack has resolved. Co-prescription with a PPI is recommended for gastroprotection. Aspirin is not indicated in gout. Oral colchicine can be used concomitantly with NSAIDs to control the attack, or alone if there is intolerance of, or side-effects to NSAIDs.

The choice of first-line agent depends on patient preference, renal function and co-morbidities. Joint aspiration and intra-articular steroids can be used as an option, especially in mono-articular cases, e.g. 1st MTP joint, which is found in >80% of cases.

Colchicine is a component of treatment for acute gout. Consider prescribing colchicine when initiating or increasing the dose of a ULT as prophylaxis against acute attacks secondary to ULT, and continue for up to 6 months. If colchicine is not tolerated, consider a low dose NSAID or coxib with gastroprotection as an alternative, provided there are no contraindications. Colchicine, which can be co-prescribed with urate-lowering therapy, has been shown to reduce episodes of gout.

If subjects cannot tolerate oral NSAIDs or colchicine, and if intra-articular injection is not possible, then a patient can be prescribed a short course of oral corticosteroids. Paracetamol can also be considered as an addition to pain relief.

Table 3.2. Treatment of acute and chronic gout (rows with light background are 1st-line therapy; those with darker background are 2nd- and 3rd-line therapy)

Drug	Formulation and dose	Mechanism of action	Usual level of therapy (NICE guidelines)	Screening	Monitoring
NSAIDs **a. Naproxen (non-COX selective)**	PO/SC Typically 250–500mg, 1–2 times per day in divided doses	Inhibition of cyclooxygenase I and II for non-COX-II selective inhibitors	1st line	Peptic ulcer disease, renal impairment, asthma	FBC, U+Es, LFTs
b. Celecoxib (COX-II selective)	Typically 200–400mg daily, 1–2 times per day in divided doses	Inhibition of COX-II for cyclooxygenase II inhibitors, e.g. etoricoxib			
Colchicine	PO Typically 500 micrograms 2–4 times daily in divided doses	Microtubule inhibitor	1st line	Exclude dehydration, previous GI problems such as diarrhoea and vomiting	FBC, U+Es
Corticosteroids, e.g. prednisolone	PO/IM/intra-articular (IA)	Works through multiple pathways, including increased transcription of anti-inflammatory genes	1st line	Monitor for diabetes, hypertension	FBC, U+Es, LFTs
Allopurinol	100–300mg PO	Xanthine oxidase inhibitor	2nd line	Renal function, uric acid	FBC, U+Es, LFTs, uric acid
Febuxostat	40–120mg PO	Xanthine oxidase inhibitor	2nd line	Renal and liver function, uric acid	FBC, U+Es, LFTs, uric acid
Anakinra	1–2mg/kg/day SC	Interleukin-1 receptor antagonist fusion protein	2nd line	Hepatitis B & C, HIV	FBC, U+Es, LFTs, uric acid
Canakinumab	150mg SC	Biologic inhibiting interleukin-1 beta receptor binding	2nd line	Hepatitis B & C, HIV	FBC, U+Es, LFTs, uric acid
Benzbromarone	50–200 mg PO	Uricosuric action	3rd line	Renal and liver function, uric acid	FBC, U+Es, LFTs, uric acid
Rasburicase	200 micrograms/kg	Enzymatic oxidation of uric acid	3rd line	Renal and liver function, uric acid, G6PD deficiency	FBC, U+Es, LFTs, uric acid
Pegloticase	8mg every 2–4 weeks	Enzymatic oxidation of uric acid	3rd line	Renal and liver function, uric acid, G6PD deficiency	FBC, U+Es, LFTs, uric acid

Biologic therapies:

- Canakinumab. An inhibitor of IL-1, canakinumab can be used as a subcutaneous injection 150mg for pain intensity in acute gout. It has been shown to be more effective than corticosteroid, in the form of 40mg triamcinolone as a subcutaneous injection. However, the drug is more expensive than other treatments for acute gout and has been linked to infections, neutropenia and thrombocytopenia.

- Anakinra. Biologic therapies targeted to the cytokine IL-1, in the form of IL-1 receptor antagonist, includes a therapy for acute gout in the acute setting when a patient may not be responding to treatment with NSAIDs, colchicine and/or corticosteroids.

None of the currently available IL-1 inhibitors, including canakinumab and anakinra, are approved and recommended by NICE. Their use in clinical settings may be influenced by cost of available agents.

Chronic gout

Treatment with DMARDs. Factors determining the initiation of ULT include two or more attacks of gout in 12 months, the presence of tophi, joint damage, chronic gouty arthritis, renal impairment, a history of urinary stones, diuretic use or a young age of onset of primary gout. In order to prevent the development of further attacks and to introduce ULT, agents such as allopurinol or febuxostat are usually added. It is usual practice to wait up to 4 weeks after an acute attack of gout has settled in order to initiate ULT. Urate-lowering drugs should not be stopped during an acute attack if the patient is already established on these drugs.

Patients often need to be advised that ULT can be lifelong and regular monitoring is required. It is possible that allopurinol and febuxostat can increase the risk of acute attacks of gout just after initiating treatment, and patients should be made aware of this before starting treatment.

- Allopurinol: this is the first-line urate-lowering treatment. Allopurinol is a xanthine oxidase inhibitor. Subjects will typically be on a dose of 100–300mg to start with. The dose can be up-titrated until the serum uric acid (SUA) is <300 micromol/L. For people with renal impairment the starting and titration dose is reduced, typically to 100mg daily (see NICE guidelines).

- Febuxostat: in cases where allopurinol has not been effective, is not tolerated or is contraindicated (e.g. in renal impairment) febuxostat can be considered as a ULT. Febuxostat also inhibits xanthine oxidase. Liver function needs to be checked prior to initiation and a low dose is started, e.g. 40–80mg. If the medication is tolerated, the dose can be increased after 4 weeks if the SUA level is >300 micromol/L. With adequate monitoring, febuxostat can be continued long-term to prevent further attacks of gout.

If a patient continues to experience further attacks of gout despite the ULTs allopurinol and febuxostat, other therapies can be considered which are usually prescribed in secondary care. These include agents such as benzbromarone and probenecid.

Enzymatic therapies. Rasburicase and pegloticase are two recombinant treatments which are licensed for the management of severe, treatment-refractory, chronic gout:
- Rasburicase, a recombinant form of urate oxidase, can be used to clear uric acid from the blood and is often used in cases where high uric acid levels require clearance, e.g. before administering chemotherapy. It has also been used in resistant cases of gout when NSAIDs, colchicine and/or corticosteroids have not been effective.
- Pegloticase, like rasburicase, converts uric acid to allantoin and helps in clearance of systemic uric acid. These therapies are contraindicated in G6PD deficiency, in which the drug can precipitate a severe haemolysis.

3.2 Pseudogout

3.2.1 Introduction

Calcium pyrophosphate deposition disease (CPPD), or pseudogout, is a common condition, affecting 4–7% of the population. It is rare below the age of 60 and often occurs in joints where there is pre-existing damage, e.g. osteoarthritis. Men and women are affected equally.

3.2.2 Diagnosis

The detection of calcium pyrophosphate (CPP) crystals under polarised light microscopy in synovial fluid aspirated from symptomatic and asymptomatic joints is required to make a firm diagnosis. CPP crystals are rhomboid-shaped and show positive birefringence under polarised light. The most commonly affected joints in CPPD include the knees and small joints of the hand, including the wrists. Since crystals can also be isolated during an asymptomatic inter-critical period, or between joint flares, a diagnosis of pseudogout can also be made in between joint flares. CPPD is often diagnosed during an intercurrent illness such as an infective episode, or joint trauma.

Plain radiographs are often performed at the time of presentation and may be normal. Other changes which can be observed include calcification, or chondrocalcinosis, in the joint space, e.g. meniscal region of the knee, triangular cartilage of the wrist, or development of 'hook-like osteophytes', due to the deposition of CPP crystals.

3.2.3 Causes

A number of risk factors are recognised for CPPD, which includes a number of metabolic disorders. These include metabolic disorders, such as hypothyroidism, primary hyperparathyroidism, acromegaly, diabetes mellitus, Wilson's disease, haemochromatosis and gout. Other rare causes of CPPD include congenital hypophosphatasia, a congenital condition that is associated with low functional levels of alkaline phosphatase.

3.2.4 Management

The management of acute CPPD is identical to that of acute gout. In the chronic phase, a focus is placed on the management and control of risk factors in order to prevent further attacks from occurring.

It is recommended that subjects presenting with no underlying case of CPPD should have iron studies, including measurement of iron, transferrin and ferritin levels, as well as measurement of levels of serum calcium, alkaline phosphatase and parathyroid hormone.

3.3 Cases

The following case histories are real-life examples demonstrating diagnosis and decision-making processes for gout management in the context of therapies available for treatment.

Case history 3.1

A 56-year-old man presented to his GP with acute onset of pain, swelling and stiffness in his right knee. He was unable to walk and had not experienced any previous episodes of this kind. The GP diagnosed acute gout and prescribed naproxen 500mg twice daily with omeprazole 30mg daily. The patient took the medication for 3 days and improved. Since he improved, the patient then went on a 10-mile walk but unfortunately was unable to complete the walk due to further swelling and pain in his knee. He attended A&E since he was unable to walk. He went on to have a knee aspiration which showed the following:

White cells >50, mainly neutrophils, no growth and abundant negatively birefringent crystals.

A diagnosis of gout was confirmed.

What treatment would you recommend?

A range of options are available:
- Intra-articular joint aspiration and injection with corticosteroid
- Alternative NSAIDs
- Oral colchicine
- All of the above

For this patient, the best option would be to aspirate the joint fully to ensure that fluid is removed. The patient can be offered a corticosteroid injection into the joint, e.g. 40mg Depo-Medrone or triamcinolone, at the same time.

Since the initial attack was probably not fully treated before the patient stopped the initial NSAIDs, he is likely to require treatment for a longer period in order to control his symptoms. A typical attack can last up to 7–10 days. He can be prescribed an NSAID and this can also be combined with colchicine, e.g. 500 mcg every 3–4 hours until the acute attack settles. The patient should be warned about the development of diarrhoea on higher doses of colchicine. The dose can be adjusted according to symptoms.

The patient's right knee swelling improves after 2 weeks and he wants advice about future treatment. Since gout has now been confirmed, he asks what he should do in future if this happens again.

What do you suggest?

- Lifestyle advice, including losing weight, reducing alcohol intake, a low purine diet
- Take NSAIDs and/or colchicine if further knee pain/swelling develops

The patient should be advised on lifestyle measures and also to take anti-inflammatories to control further attacks. If his symptoms settle and his uric acid level is in the normal range, he does not require ULT, but can be monitored in the GP surgery.

Case history 3.2

A 65-year-old man presents to his GP with bilateral foot pain in both big toes. He has been unable to walk as a result of his symptoms for the last few days. He has taken paracetamol with no major relief. He has a significant past medical history of diabetes mellitus, hypertension and renal tract stones. He is on gliclazide, amlodipine and has recently been started on furosemide as his blood pressure has been difficult to control.

His GP does some urgent blood tests, which show the following:
- Na 136
- K 4.6
- Urea 9.4
- Creat 106
- Urate 601
- Glucose 9.9

The GP diagnoses acute gout.

He prescribes colchicine 500 micrograms every 3–4 hours. He warns the patient that he may develop GI side-effects such as abdominal pain and diarrhoea. Unfortunately, the patient is unable to tolerate the medication as he develops diarrhoea.

What do you prescribe to manage his foot pain?

Prednisolone 30mg on a dose reducing by 5mg every 3 days is prescribed to control the patient's acute attack. This is because he cannot have NSAIDs as a result of his renal impairment and he was unable to tolerate colchicine.

Two months later the man is admitted to hospital with renal colic. A kidney, ureter and bladder X-ray confirms that that he has a calculus in his right kidney. He passes the stone and it is confirmed to contain uric acid.

What treatment do you recommend?

The patient requires ULT. Since he has renal impairment, he needs to be given a lower starting dose, e.g. allopurinol 100mg daily.

He will require monitoring of his SUA levels to see if they come down with treatment, and also his renal function requires monitoring 4–6 weeks after initiating treatment and then 3–6-monthly.

He remains compliant with medication and experiences a reduction in episodes of gout and renal colic.

Since renal tract stones are a recognised complication of gout, it is important to ensure that ULT is started early to prevent the development of long-term complications such as renal tract stones, joint erosions and gouty tophi.

Case history 3.3

A 75-year-old woman presents with acute pain and swelling of her right knee. On examination there is reduced range of movement with a positive patellar tap. She is overweight. There is no history of previous trauma, joint pain or swelling.

What is the single most important investigation?

- Aspiration of knee joint synovial fluid
- Serum urate
- Blood cultures
- CRP measurement
- Serum RhF

The patient needs a knee joint synovial fluid aspiration because the differential diagnosis includes gout, CPPD, an acute flare of osteoarthritis or septic arthritis.

The patient is in pain. Her other medications include amlodipine for hypertension.

What would be the first treatment of choice?

- Oral corticosteroids
- Ibuprofen
- Codeine phosphate
- Morphine sulphate
- Amitriptyline

In the absence of side-effects and renal impairment, an NSAID would be the first choice for the management of acute CPPD.

The patient goes on to have a joint aspiration, with removal of 40ml of straw-coloured fluid, which is sent for urgent Gram stain. Plain X-rays show osteoarthritis and chondrocalcinosis with linear calcification along the joint margin. Knee aspirate confirms the presence of calcium pyrophosphate crystals.

An X-ray is taken, showing knee joint space narrowing and sclerosis, and linear calcification (shown by arrows) indicating chondrocalcinosis.

Anteroposterior view   **Lateral view**

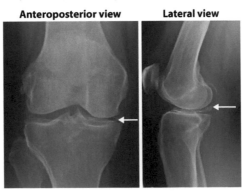

3.4 References

Bardin, T., Bouée, S., Clerson, P. *et al.* (2016) Prevalence of gout in the adult population of France. *Arthritis Care Res.*, **68(2)**: 261–6.

Hui, M., Carr, A., Cameron, S. *et al.* (2017) The British Society for Rheumatology Guideline for the Management of Gout. *Rheumatology*, **56(7)**: e1–e20.

Kuo, C-F., Grainge, M.J., See, L-C. *et al.* (2015a) Epidemiology and management of gout in Taiwan: a nationwide population study. *Arthritis Res Ther.*, **17(1)**: 13.

Kuo, C-F., Grainge, M.J., Mallen, C. *et al.* (2015b) Rising burden of gout in the UK but continuing suboptimal management: a nationwide population study. *Ann Rheum Dis.*, **74(4)**: 661–667.

Richette, P., Doherty, M., Pascual, E. *et al.* (2020) 2018 updated European League Against Rheumatism evidence-based recommendations for the diagnosis of gout. *Ann Rheum Dis.*, **79(1)**: 31–38.

Rosenthal, A.K. and Ryan, L.M. (2016) Calcium pyrophosphate deposition disease. *NEJM*, **374(26)**: 2575–2584.

Zhu, Y., Pandya, B.J. and Choi, H.K. (2011) Prevalence of gout and hyperuricemia in the US general population: the National Health and Nutrition Examination survey 2007–2008. *Arthritis Rheum.*, **63(10)**: 3136–41.

NICE and BSR guidelines

NICE guidelines for the management of gout
https://cks.nice.org.uk/gout
www.nice.org.uk/guidance/TA164

BSR guidelines
https://academic.oup.com/rheumatology/article/55/9/1693/1744535

Psoriatic arthritis

04

4.1 Introduction

Psoriatic arthritis (PsA) is a condition with a prevalence of 10–30% of people affected by psoriasis. The prevalence of psoriasis of the skin is estimated at 2–3% in the general population. PsA can affect a young age range of people, with a peak onset from 30 up to 50 years. Arthritic involvement is usually preceded by psoriasis which affects the skin. Men tend to develop axial disease, with women developing peripheral joint involvement more frequently. Other factors influencing the development of PsA include genetic susceptibility and infection (*Figure 4.1*). Interestingly, some people with arthritic involvement may not have previously had significant cutaneous involvement. It is not fully understood why certain people with psoriasis develop PsA.

4.2 Diagnosis

Symptoms of PsA include joint stiffness, swelling, pain and fatigue. All the symptoms described can make day-to-day activities difficult, and cause pain and functional impairment. PsA can have serious effects on the skin and joints, resulting in a serious negative effect on people's quality of life. PsA can affect people from a young age, and it can affect multiple aspects of people's lives, including their family life, relationships and career aspirations. The psychological impact of the condition is significant.

4.2.1 Features of psoriatic arthritis

Joints

There are different forms of joint involvement in psoriatic arthritis. Joint involvement can be limited to a few joints only, e.g. peripheral small joints of the hands, while in other cases there can be more extensive involvement. Classically there are five different forms of PsA involvement:

- Symmetric small joint involvement – this form is similar to an RA distribution
- Asymmetric large joint involvement – predominantly large joints are involved in this form, e.g. knee or foot
- Peripheral small joint involvement – the distal interphalangeal joints are predominantly involved
- Axial spondyloarthritis – in this form there is mainly spinal disease, with possible enthesitis, bone oedema and/or sacroiliitis
- Arthritis mutilans – this is a very severe form of the disease which can lead to complete destruction of the joint, with changes such as telescoping of the fingers and severe loss of function.

Psoriatic arthritis is typified by several other clinical features which are not usually observed in other inflammatory arthritides such as RA.

More recently, it has been recommended that the diagnosis of psoriatic arthritis is made based on the CASPAR criteria, which include the following:

CASPAR criteria

- Inflammatory arthritic disease
- Current, personal or family history of psoriasis
- Psoriatic nail dystrophy
- Negative test for RhF
- Dactylitis: current swelling of entire digit, or history of dactylitis
- Radiologic evidence of juxta-articular new bone formation.

Tendinitis

Inflammation of the tendons is a feature of PsA. Tendinopathies can occur in any part of the body.

Enthesitis

This is inflammation of the entheses, which is where ligaments or tendons insert into bones. The most frequent areas of enthesitis include the feet, the Achilles tendon, and attachments to the ribs, spine and pelvis. Over a longer period of time, ongoing enthesitis can lead to fibrosis (or thickening of the enthesites), calcification or ossification. Enthesitis is not usually observed in rheumatoid arthritis and osteoarthritis.

Dactylitis

This is commonly known as 'sausage digits', and is a result of inflammation in the whole finger or toe. Dactylitis occurs when small joints and entheses of the surrounding tendons become inflamed. Dactylitis is a typical hallmark of PsA. It can involve a few fingers or toes but is usually asymmetrical. PsA can affect different toes and fingers on either side.

Skin and nails

Psoriatic skin changes are often typified by a scaly, maculopapular rash at the extensor surfaces of the body, e.g. elbows, hairline and umbilicus. In more severe cases, it can be increasingly widespread and cover large areas of the body.

The degree of skin involvement does not always correlate with the extent of joint involvement. If there is severe skin disease that requires treatment with disease-modifying therapy, it is sometimes possible that skin and joints can be treated together with DMARDs.

Nails can show features of ridging, pitting and onycholysis. These can be found early and may be present in the absence of more widespread cutaneous involvement.

4.2.2 Investigations

Blood tests

Psoriatic arthritis is a seronegative arthritis, which means that autoantibody screening is usually negative, including ANA, RhF and anti-CCP. The patient may have raised inflammatory markers, including ESR and CRP. The HLA-B27 tends to be negative in PsA and is a more prominent feature of ankylosing spondylitis.

Imaging

Plain radiographs may show erosions if the arthritis is established and there has been bone destruction. Ultrasound may be useful in

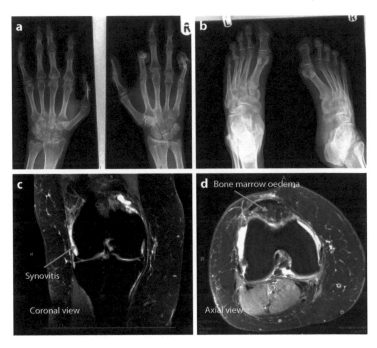

Figure 4.1. Examples of radiographic changes observed in psoriatic arthritis

(a) Plain radiographs of the hand showing erosions and joint space narrowing in distal interphalangeal joints, proximal interphalangeal joints and metacarpophalangeal joints of both hands. The patient has had surgery in the left thumb, right index and little fingers. There is also wrist involvement with fusion of the carpal bones in the left wrist and erosions in the right wrist. (b) Plain radiographs of the feet in the same patient as in part (a). There is bone loss, erosions and joint deviation as a result of long-term damage. (c) MRI scan of the knee in a patient with PsA of the knee. The T1 weighted image shows synovitis as high signal on MRI, consistent with inflammation (green arrow). (d) MRI scan of the knee in the same patient as in part (c). The axial view shows bone marrow oedema in the patella (green arrow).

demonstrating synovitis with increased power Doppler signal and early erosions. Such changes may assist in supporting the need to commence DMARDs. More recently, MRI has been used and can be helpful in detecting enthesitis and also bone marrow oedema. Examples of imaging changes observed in PsA are summarised in *Figure 4.1*.

4.3 Causes

Risk factors for PsA include genetics. Having a parent with psoriasis triples the chance of developing psoriasis. *Figure 4.2* shows a

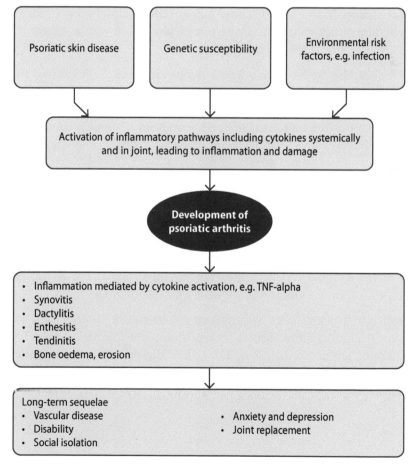

Figure 4.2. The development of psoriatic arthritis

summary of the development of PsA. Epidemiology suggests that there is a strong genetic contribution in PsA. There are some genetic differences between people with skin and joint involvement. Coding variants are described in TYK2 and TRAF3IP2, which are strongly associated with skin and joint disease. Some studies have focused on biomarkers for PsA, showing that genomics and serological factors may play a role in treatment response to TNF inhibitors. Infections such as streptococcal throat can also be associated with the development of PsA.

4.4 Management

The treatment of PsA often involves a multidisciplinary approach, which includes treatment of the joint and skin, as well as physical, social and psychological factors.

For skin, the extent of cutaneous involvement can be measured by the Psoriasis Area and Severity Index (PASI), which is a composite score of body surface area, erythema, induration, and scaling of psoriasis on different areas of the body (head, trunk, upper limbs, lower limbs). It is mainly used in clinical trials as it can take significant time to measure in clinic.

A wide range of joints can be affected in PsA, therefore a scoring system needs to reflect that. In the clinic, patients are often shown mannequins to measure the extent of joint involvement when they are assessed (*Figure 4.3*). The Psoriatic Arthritis Response Criteria (PsARC) score is used quite extensively in clinical settings, with the number of tender and swollen joints recorded and used with a range of scoring from 1 (mild disease) to 5 (severe disease).

Recently, clinical trials are including a range of disease activity scores in psoriatic arthritis, among them the Psoriatic ArthritiS Disease Activity Score (PASDAS), the GRAppa Composite score (GRACE index) and the Composite Psoriatic Disease Activity Index (CPDAI).

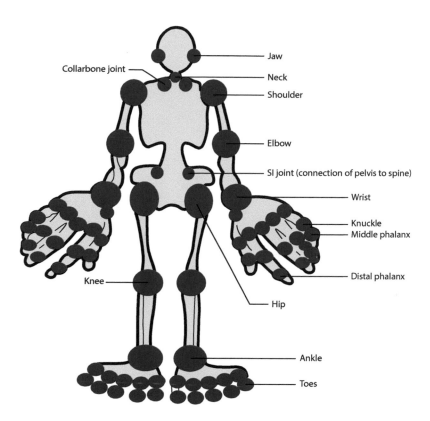

Figure 4.3. Example of mannequin used to assess joints in psoriatic arthritis

4.4.1 Non-pharmacological therapies

Physiotherapy has a role to play in strengthening joint structures and helping to maintain function. People may also require occupational therapy, e.g. for hand supports and splinting, and psychological support may be needed in cases where the mental health impact of psoriasis and arthritis plays a part.

4.4.2 Pharmacological management

A summary of the principles of pharmacological management in PsA is given in *Table 4.1*.

Table 4.1. Pharmacological management of psoriatic arthritis as per NICE guidelines (rows with light background show drugs used 1st line; those with darker background are biologic agents used as 2nd-line therapies)

Drug	Formulation and dose	Mechanism of action	Usual level of therapy (NICE guidelines)	Screening	Monitoring
Methotrexate	PO/SC Typically 15–25mg weekly	Inhibition of purine synthesis	1st line	Hepatitis B & C, HIV	FBC, U+Es, LFTs
Sulfasalazine	PO Typically 2–3g daily	Inhibition of expression of TNF and other cytokines	1st line	Hepatitis B & C, HIV	FBC, U+Es, LFTs
Leflunomide	PO Typically 20mg daily after loading dose	Inhibition of pyrimidine synthesis	1st line	Hepatitis B & C, HIV	FBC, U+Es, LFTs
Hydroxychloroquine	PO Up to 400mg daily in divided doses	Inhibition of expression of TNF and other cytokines	1st line	Hepatitis B & C, HIV	FBC, U+Es, LFTs
Corticosteroids, e.g. prednisolone	PO/IM/IA/topical	Works through multiple pathways including increased transcription of anti-inflammatory genes	1st line	Monitor for diabetes, hypertension	
Apremilast	PO Up to 30mg twice daily	Phosphodiesterase 4 (PDE4) inhibitor	1st to 2nd line NICE TA433	Hepatitis B & C, HIV	FBC, U+Es, LFTs
Infliximab (Remicade/ Remsima biosimilar)	IV 0-, 2-, 6- then 8-weekly	Chimeric anti-TNF monoclonal antibody	2nd line NICE TA199	Hepatitis B & C, HIV, TB	FBC, U+Es, LFTs
Adalimumab (Humira)	40mg SC every 2 weeks	Humanised anti-TNF monoclonal antibody	2nd line NICE TA199	Hepatitis B & C, HIV, TB	FBC, U+Es, LFTs

	Dose	Mechanism	Line / NICE	Screening	Monitoring
Etanercept (Enbrel, Benepali biosimilar)	50mg SC weekly or 25mg twice weekly	TNF fusion protein	2nd line NICE TA199	Hepatitis B & C, HIV, TB	FBC, U+Es, LFTs
Certolizumab	200mg every 2 weeks or 400mg every 4 weeks	Pegylated TNF antibody	2nd line NICE TA445	Hepatitis B & C, HIV, TB	FBC, U+Es, LFTs
Golimumab	50mg monthly. Consider 100mg monthly in those >100kg if inadequate response at 50mg	Humanised anti-TNF monoclonal antibody	2nd line NICE TA220	Hepatitis B & C, HIV, TB	FBC, U+Es, LFTs
Secukinumab	150mg monthly	Humanised monoclonal antibody to IL-17A	2nd line NICE TA445	Hepatitis B & C, HIV, TB	FBC, U+Es, LFTs
Ustekinumab	45mg every 12 weeks, or 90mg every 12 weeks in those >100kg requiring higher dose	Monoclonal antibody targeting IL-12 and IL-23	2nd line NICE TA340	Hepatitis B & C, HIV, TB	FBC, U+Es, LFTs
Ixekizumab	80mg 4-weekly	Humanised monoclonal antibody to IL-17A	2nd line NICE TA537	Hepatitis B & C, HIV, TB	FBC, U+Es, LFTs
Tofacitinib	5mg twice daily	JAK inhibitor	2nd line NICE TA543	Hepatitis B & C, HIV, TB	FBC, U+Es, LFTs Lipids Monitor for herpes zoster

In the initial stages, NSAIDs can be used to treat joint stiffness, swelling and pain. For flare-ups, or the injection of one joint (e.g. the knee), which may have flared, corticosteroids can be used. A typical oral dose for a flare may be 20–40mg daily on a reducing dose. For intramuscular injections, typical doses range from 80–120mg. For intra-articular injections, doses range from 40–80mg of Depo-Medrone or triamcinolone.

Disease-modifying antirheumatic drugs

In order to prevent long-term damage to the joints and to control skin involvement, DMARD therapies have been used, backed up by clinical trials.

Oral synthetic DMARDs are considered to be the first-line agents for control of PsA and often also have a beneficial effect on the joints. They include methotrexate, sulfasalazine and apremilast.

In patients where oral synthetic DMARDs have been ineffective in providing optimal disease control, biologic agents have been licensed and approved by NICE and are used. These include adalimumab, certolizumab, etanercept, golimumab, infliximab, secukinumab, ustekinumab, ixekizumab and tofacitinib.

4.5 Cases

The following cases are based on real patients and are presented to help you consider how you would manage the scenarios.

Case history 4.1

A 25-year-old man presented with a swollen knee. He developed the swelling without any trauma or injury. He developed psoriasis in his late teens but was otherwise well. He was referred urgently to the rheumatologist. On examination, he had a large joint effusion in his right knee. The rheumatologist aspirated the knee to obtain 15ml of straw-coloured fluid. The fluid was sent for microscopy, culture and sensitivity. The aspirate returned no growth or crystals. There was a mixed population of white cells with neutrophils and macrophages seen.

Further blood tests showed a negative ANA, rheumatoid factor and anti-CCP antibodies. His CRP was increased at 22ng/ml and the ESR was 34mm/hr.

What would you prescribe for his knee pain?

- Naproxen 500mg bd
- Naproxen 500mg bd with omeprazole 20mg daily
- Prednisolone 40mg orally daily for 1 week
- Codeine phosphate 30mg as required
- Paracetamol 1g four times daily

An NSAID would be indicated, with a PPI, to control the inflammation. High dose prednisolone would normally be given if more than one joint was involved. The patient could also be offered intra-articular corticosteroid if they wished. Codeine is not helpful for inflammatory pain in acute psoriatic arthritis. Paracetamol is unlikely to be effective.

The patient improved for a few weeks but unfortunately returned 6 weeks later with more pain, stiffness and swelling involving both knees, with dactylitis in his toes of both feet.

What would be the next treatment option?

- Start prednisolone and consider starting methotrexate
- Methotrexate alone
- Further course of NSAIDs
- Consider starting biologic anti-TNF therapy
- Switch to another type of NSAID

The patient has developed more extensive disease and requires control of the acute episode with corticosteroids and then longer-term DMARD medication in the form of methotrexate, which is first line. A further course of steroids is unlikely to control recurrent episodes and the patient is likely to require more long-term DMARD therapy. The patient requires a trial of synthetic DMARDs, such as methotrexate, before starting biologic therapy, as directed by NICE guidelines. Switching to another DMARD is unlikely to provide optimal disease control.

The patient is started on a course of oral prednisolone 20mg on a reducing dose and is also counselled for methotrexate, which he starts at 15mg weekly, and folic acid 5mg weekly. His knee swelling becomes better controlled and his dactylitis also improves. He stays on methotrexate and remains in remission, with regular review and blood monitoring.

Case history 4.2

A 45-year-old man has a long-standing history of PsA. He has had surgery, including PIP joint surgeries, but is flaring. He has previously tried multiple courses of prednisolone for joint flares and is also on methotrexate DMARD therapy 15mg weekly. He is considered for second-line biologic therapy. At his screening visit, he reports to the nurse that he has a strong family history of multiple sclerosis (MS).

What agents can he be considered for, to control his psoriatic arthritis?

- Adalimumab
- Tocilizumab
- Ustekinumab
- Secukinumab
- Tofacitinib

The patient would be considered high risk for developing multiple sclerosis from TNF inhibitor therapy, which is a known risk factor for MS. Therefore, he should be counselled and considered for alternative biologic therapies to anti-TNF treatments, which include the IL-12/23 inhibitors such as ustekinumab, the IL-17A inhibitors such as secukinumab, ixekinumab and the JAK inhibitor tofacitinib. A decision is often made together with the patient, based on providing information about benefits and potential side-effects, ease of use (e.g. oral versus injection) and patient preference. For example, a patient who prefers oral therapy may be better suited to tofacitinib rather than injection therapies such as ustekinumab, secukinumab or ixekinumab. Due to the variety of treatments available, if a patient does not achieve an improvement after 12 weeks of one agent, they can then be considered for an alternative second-line therapy.

4.6 References

Gossec, L., Smolen, J.S., Ramiro, S. *et al.* (2016) European League Against Rheumatism (EULAR) recommendations for the management of psoriatic arthritis with pharmacological therapies: 2015 update. *Ann Rheum Dis.*, **75(3)**: 499–510.

Helliwell, P.S., FitzGerald, O., Fransen, J. *et al.* (2013) The development of candidate composite disease activity and responder indices for psoriatic arthritis (GRACE project). *Ann Rheum Dis.*, **72(6)**: 986–991.

Orbai, A-M., de Wit, M., Mease, P. *et al.* (2017) International patient and physician consensus on a psoriatic arthritis core outcome set for clinical trials. *Ann Rheum Dis.*, **76(4)**: 673–680.

NICE, BSR guidelines and useful websites

Coates, L.C., Tillett, W., Chandler, D. *et al.* (2013) The 2012 BSR and BHPR guideline for the treatment of psoriatic arthritis with biologics. *Rheumatology*, **52(10)**: 1754–1757.

Group for Research and Assessment of Psoriasis and Psoriatic Arthritis: www. grappanetwork.org/

NICE guidelines: www.nice.org.uk/search?q=Psoriatic+arthritis

05

Ankylosing spondylitis

5.1 Introduction

Ankylosing spondylitis (AS) is a long-term condition, predominantly affecting the spine. The axial skeleton is the focus of inflammation, which can flare on different occasions. The prevalence of AS is 0.1–0.5% in populations worldwide. The most common age of AS presentation is in younger people, particularly in teenagers and young adults, ranging in age from twenties to thirties. It is approximately twice as common in men than in women.

5.2 Diagnosis

The symptoms of AS include back pain and stiffness, which typically shows a diurnal variation that is worse in the mornings. Symptoms of early morning stiffness focused around the spine and/or sacroiliac joints are a recognised feature of the inflammatory back pain due to AS. Sustained pain of at least 3 months, which is relieved by exercise and not by rest, is a characteristic feature. Limitation of spinal movements in the frontal and sagittal planes is also characteristic. Pain and swelling in other regions may also be found, including at sites where tendons insert into bone, e.g. Achilles tendinitis.

Some patients also experience inflammation in the eye, including uveitis, scleritis and episcleritis. Although more rare, peripheral joint involvement can also be found. Since AS is a multisystem condition, there can be involvement of the vascular system (e.g. aortic regurgitation) and lung involvement, with pulmonary fibrosis.

Patients need to be monitored closely to prevent the progression and for early treatment of extra-articular involvement, to prevent long-term complications.

Any suspected cases of inflammatory back pain should be referred promptly to assist with early diagnosis and treatment. Clinical assessment includes a number of measurements, such as wall-to-tragus distance, chest expansion and a modified Schober's test to test flexion of the spine. Baseline measurements are important and these can be tracked as the patient is monitored over time with treatments including physiotherapy and pharmacological interventions.

Important clinical features assisting in the diagnosis of AS:
- early morning stiffness features of spinal pain
- symptoms improve with exercise
- improves with NSAIDs
- presence of HLA-B27 positivity on blood testing
- spinal disease more frequent in men, peripheral disease more frequent in women.

Various diagnostic criteria have been developed in the last decade. The Assessment of SpondyloArthritis international Society (ASAS) has developed criteria for the diagnosis of axial and peripheral joint disease, summarised below.

For axial disease, in subjects under the age of 45 with more than 3 months of back pain, axial spondyloarthritis can be diagnosed by the presence of sacroiliitis on imaging and one or more features of the following: inflammatory back pain, arthritis, enthesitis (heel), uveitis, dactylitis, psoriasis, Crohn's disease/colitis, good clinical response to NSAIDs, family history of SpA, HLA-B27 and an elevated CRP. For subjects who are HLA-B27 positive, two or more features described above are required to make a diagnosis of axial spondyloarthritis. The criteria are reported to have a sensitivity of 82.9% and specificity of 84.4%. Blood testing may show some evidence of inflammation, including ESR and CRP. Testing blood for the genetic haplotype HLA-B27 allele is useful since it can assist with confirming diagnosis and future management. Autoantibodies including ANA, RhF and anti-CCP antibodies are typically negative in AS.

In recent years, imaging has become important in the diagnosis and ongoing management of AS. Most subjects will now undergo screening of the whole spine and sacroiliac joints by MRI with short T1 inversion recovery (STIR) sequences. Characteristic changes on MRI include synovitis, enthesitis or capsulitis without bone oedema or osteitis. Other structural changes that are found radiographically in AS include erosions, fat deposits, sclerosis or ankyloses. (Examples of radiographic changes are shown in *Case histories 5.1* and *5.2*.)

Since AS often presents with back pain, it is important to check for red flags in any patient with back pain, as follows:

Red flags for back pain

Any 'red flags' highlighted during an assessment need urgent referral. These include the following:
- acute cord injury or disc prolapse
- suspected tumour or malignancy (urgent referral following the local 2-week cancer referral pathway)
- suspected joint infection
- acute fracture as a result of trauma
- back pain with symptoms suggestive of a systemic inflammatory joint disease should be referred to Rheumatology via local referral pathways.

5.3 Causes

Genetic background is a known risk factor in AS. The HLA-B27 allele is found in approximately up to 90% of cases, but only in 8% of the general white population. The development of AS is summarised in *Figure 5.1*. In the UK, HLA-B27 is found in 90–95% of people who have a diagnosis of AS, in 60–90% of patients with reactive arthritis, and in 50–60% of patients with PsA or inflammatory bowel disease and spondylitis. Several theories have been proposed to explain how HLA-B27 might predispose to spondyloarthritis. For example, HLA-B27 is capable of presenting potentially arthritogenic peptides to cytotoxic T lymphocytes. Molecular mimicry has also been described between an amino acid sequence in HLA-B*2705 and products of the pathogens *Klebsiella* and *Shigella*. HLA-B27 also enhances the invasion of *Salmonella* into intestinal epithelial cells.

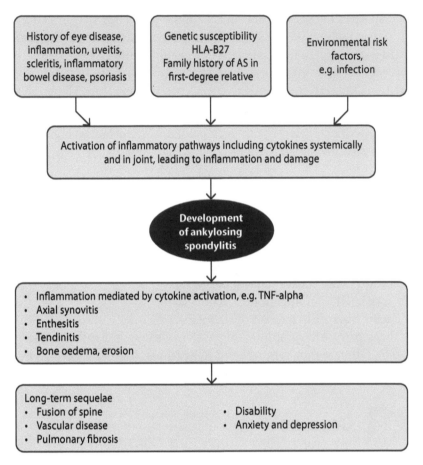

Figure 5.1. The development of ankylosing spondylitis

The microbiome is also thought to play a role in the development of AS, particularly with gut exposure to particular pathogens. In spondyloarthritis, it has been suggested that dysbiosis with altered gut bacteria influences intestinal permeability and intestinal immune responses. The presence of intestinal dysbiosis is found in people with spondyloarthritis which can lead to changes in gut–epithelial and gut–vascular barriers. The leakage of epithelial and endothelial surface layers is followed by the translocation of bacterial products, such as lipopolysaccharide and intestinal fatty acid binding protein into the circulation. In the gut, IL-23 is thought to induce expansion of immune cells such as different types of T cells and lymphoid cells.

There is also a recognised overlap between the development of AS and inflammatory bowel disease, inflammation of the eye and psoriasis (see *Chapter 4*). All these risk factors should be screened for when taking a patient's history.

5.4 Management

Initial education about the condition and maintaining physical activity is important. Physiotherapy is recommended as it is helpful to alleviate inflammatory joint symptoms. Pharmacological therapies also play an important role, as many patients are young at first diagnosis and are likely to require multiple treatments over a long period of time. The level of pain and function can be monitored using the spinal Visual Analogue Scale (VAS) score in clinic and the Bath Ankylosing Spondylitis Disease Activity Index (BASDAI).

5.4.1 Non-pharmacological management

Physiotherapy

Refer patients to a specialist physiotherapist to start an individualised, structured exercise programme, consisting of stretching, strengthening and postural exercises. In addition deep breathing exercises, range of motion exercises for the lumbar, thoracic and cervical spine are recommended. Regular aerobic exercise is also important. Hydrotherapy can also be used as an adjunct therapy to manage pain and improve function. Further information about exercise is provided in *Chapter 10*. The National Axial Spondyloarthritis Society (NASS) (nass.co.uk) is also helpful in providing information about local groups. Exercises focused on breathing and maintaining posture and flexibility of the spine are important. The importance of regular physical activity to maintain motion is also stressed.

5.4.2 Pharmacological treatment

Treatment options include NSAIDs in the initial phases of AS, followed by maintenance of disease control with DMARDs (shown in *Table 5.1*).

Table 5.1. Disease-modifying drugs for AS (drugs in rows with light background can be used for peripheral joint involvement and can be used as 1st line; biologic therapies in rows with darker background can be used as 2nd line when NSAIDs and/or synthetic DMARDs have not been effective)

Drug	Formulation and dose	Mechanism of action	Usual level of therapy (NICE guidelines)	Screening	Monitoring
NSAIDs • Naproxen (non-COX selective) • Celecoxib (COX-II selective)	PO/SC Typically 250–500mg, 1–2 times per day in divided doses Typically 200–400mg daily, 1–2 times per day in divided doses	Inhibition of cyclooxygenase I and II for non-COX-II selective inhibitors Inhibition of COX-II for cyclooxygenase II inhibitors, e.g. etoricoxib	1st line	Peptic ulcer disease, renal impairment, asthma	FBC, U+Es, LFTs
Methotrexate	PO/SC Typically 15–25mg weekly	Inhibition of purine synthesis	1st line	Hepatitis B & C, HIV	FBC, U+Es, LFTs
Leflunomide	PO Typically 20mg daily after loading dose	Inhibition of pyrimidine synthesis	1st line	Hepatitis B & C, HIV	FBC, U+Es, LFTs
Azathioprine	PO Typically 50–150mg daily in divided doses	Inhibition of purine synthesis	1st line	Hepatitis B & C, HIV	FBC, U+Es, LFTs
Sulfasalazine	PO Typically 1–3g daily in divided doses	Inhibitor of expression of TNF and other cytokines	1st line	Hepatitis B & C, HIV	FBC, U+Es, LFTs
Hydroxychloroquine	PO Up to 400mg daily in divided doses	Inhibitor of expression of TNF and other cytokines	1st line	Hepatitis B & C, HIV	FBC, U+Es, LFTs
Corticosteroids, e.g. prednisolone	PO/IM	Works through multiple pathways including increased transcription of anti-inflammatory genes	1st line	Monitor for diabetes, hypertension	FBC, U+Es, LFTs

Infliximab (Remicade/ Remsima biosimilar)	IV 0-, 2-, 6- then 8-weekly	Chimeric anti-TNF monoclonal antibody	2nd line	Hepatitis B & C, HIV	FBC, U+Es, LFTs
Adalimumab (Humira)	40mg SC every 2 weeks	Humanised anti-TNF monoclonal antibody	2nd line	Hepatitis B & C, HIV	FBC, U+Es, LFTs
Etanercept (Enbrel, Benepali biosimilar)	50mg SC weekly or 25mg twice weekly	TNF fusion protein	2nd line	Hepatitis B & C, HIV, TB	FBC, U+Es, LFTs
Certolizumab	200mg every 2 weeks or 400mg every 4 weeks	Pegylated TNF antibody	2nd line	Hepatitis B & C, HIV, TB	FBC, U+Es, LFTs
Golimumab	50mg monthly Consider 100mg monthly in subjects >100kg if inadequate response at 50mg	Humanised anti-TNF monoclonal antibody	2nd line	Hepatitis B & C, HIV, TB	FBC, U+Es, LFTs
Secukinumab	150mg monthly	Humanised monoclonal antibody to IL-17A	2nd line	Hepatitis B, C, HIV, TB	FBC, U+Es, LFTs

NSAIDs

According to NICE guidelines, it is recommended that NSAIDs are used for 3–6 months in the initial phases to help manage pain and inflammation. The mechanism of action of NSAIDs is by suppression of cyclooxygenase metabolites. A characteristic feature of AS is a therapeutic response to NSAIDs. It is recommended that if one type of NSAID is not effective after 3 months at the maximum dose, the patient can be switched to an alternative agent. The most commonly prescribed NSAIDs are summarised in *Table 5.1*.

DMARDs

If patients continue to experience symptoms of pain, stiffness and/ or swelling despite two different types of NSAIDs, they can be considered for DMARD agents, as summarised in *Table 5.1*. For peripheral non-axial joint involvement, oral synthetic DMARDs such as methotrexate, sulfasalazine and other agents can be considered. Biologic DMARDs are reserved for the treatment of axial disease and conventional synthetic DMARDs are not used for spinal symptoms due to lack of efficacy.

5.5 Cases

The following cases are based on real patients and are presented to help you consider how you would manage the scenarios.

Case history 5.1

A 25-year-old woman who has experienced lower back and sacroiliac pain is referred to the Rheumatologist. She used to do gymnastics and dance as a teenager, and attributed her lower back pain to those physical activities. She has tenderness in both sacroiliac joints on clinical assessment. The Rheumatologist assesses her and arranges X-rays, as shown below.

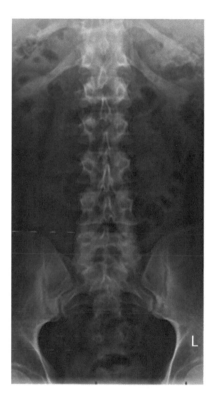

What does the radiograph show?

- Ankylosis of the lumbar vertebrae
- Periarticular sclerosis of the sacroiliac joints
- A fracture of L5
- No abnormalities
- Osteopenia of the lumbar vertebrae

The radiograph shows periarticular sclerosis of the sacroiliac joints bilaterally, which is indicative of previous joint inflammation at the sacroiliac joints. According to ASAS grading for damage to the sacroiliac joints in ankylosing spondylitis, severity can be graded from 0–4:

Grade 0   normal

Grade 1   suspicious changes

Grade 2   minimal definite changes: circumscribed areas of erosions or sclerosis with no changes of the sacroiliac joint space

Grade 3   distinctive changes, sclerosis, change of joint space (decreased or widened), partial ankylosis (fusion of the joint)

Grade 4   ankylosis

The radiographic findings are discussed with the patient and she is referred for physiotherapy. This results in a significant improvement in her back pain. She only requires NSAIDs once or twice per week. She is monitored and remains stable.

Case history 5.2

A 30-year-old man was diagnosed with AS aged 18. At that stage he had severe lower back pain and a history of psoriasis, and was HLA-B27 positive. He now works as an accountant and his job involves frequent business trips. He has stopped playing tennis and is concerned that he is finding it difficult to do his job. He is seen by the Rheumatologist, who discovers that he has taken several different NSAIDs prescribed by his GP, including naproxen, ibuprofen and diclofenac. He has also developed peptic ulcer disease as a result of chronic NSAID use, and is taking regular PPIs in the form of omeprazole.

On examination he has a reduced chest expansion of 2cm and flexion at his spine is limited to 3.5cm with a modified Schober's test. The Rheumatologist arranges an MRI scan of the whole spine to assess his level of disease activity.

The results of the MRI scan of the whole spine and pelvis are shown below:

Sagittal MRI of cervical spine

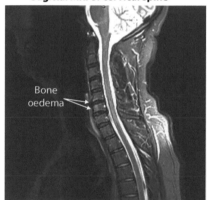

Sagittal MRI of lumbosacral spine

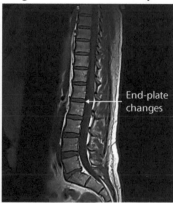

Axial MRI of sacroiliac joints

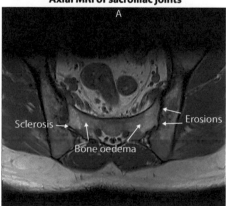

What treatment would you advise next?

- Switch to a different NSAID
- Physiotherapy
- Stop all medication and monitor the patient
- Prescribe high dose steroids
- Counsel the patient for starting anti-TNF therapy

The patient has already tried multiple different NSAIDs and has features of inflammation including bone oedema, erosions and sclerosis at the axial spine and sacroiliac joints. He qualifies for treatment with biologic drugs, as summarised in *Table 5.1*.

5.6 References

Dougados, M. and Baeten, D. (2011) Spondyloarthritis. *Lancet*, **377:** 2127–37.

Sieper, J., Rudwaleit, M., Baraliakos, X. et al. (2009) The Assessment of SpondyloArthritis international Society (ASAS) handbook: a guide to assess spondyloarthritis. *Ann Rheum Dis.*, **68(suppl 2):** ii1–ii4.

Stolwijk, C., van Tubergen, A., Castillo-Ortiz, J.D. and Boonen, A. (2015) Prevalence of extra-articular manifestations in patients with ankylosing spondylitis: a systematic review and meta-analysis. *Ann Rheum Dis.*, **74(1):** 65–73.

van der Heijde, D., Ramiro, S., Landewé, R. et al. (2017) 2016 update of the ASAS–EULAR management recommendations for axial spondyloarthritis. *Ann Rheum Dis.*, **76(6):** 978–991.

NICE, BSR guidelines and useful websites

Bath Ankylosing Spondylitis Disease Activity Index: basdai.com

British Society for Rheumatology guidelines:

Hamilton, L., Barkham, N., Bhalla, A. et al. (2017) BSR and BHPR guideline for the treatment of axial spondyloarthritis (including ankylosing spondylitis) with biologics. *Rheumatology*, **56(2):** 313–316.

Assessment of SpondyloArthritis international Society (ASAS) handbook: www.asas-group.org/education/asas-handbook

NICE guidance for physiotherapy: www.nice.org.uk/guidance/ng65/chapter/recommendations

NICE guidelines for ankylosing spondylitis pharmacological management: www.nice.org.uk/search?q=ankylosing%20spondylitis

National Axial Spondyloarthritis Society: https://nass.co.uk

CHAPTER 6

Vasculitis

6.1　Introduction

Vasculitis includes a broad range of heterogeneous conditions, all of which are characterised by abnormalities in blood vessels that are autoimmune-mediated. The overall prevalence is estimated at 1–20 per million, depending on the type of vasculitis involved. The age of onset for vasculitides is classically above 50 years. Overall across the different forms of vasculitis, male to female ratio is fairly equal. However, some forms of vasculitis are more prevalent in women, e.g. lupus nephritis, whereas other forms are more common in men, e.g. anti-neutrophil cytoplasmic antibody (ANCA)-associated vasculitis. Changes in affected blood vessels can lead to localised end-organ tissue damage that is specific in different forms of vasculitis. Classically, clinical features and histological changes on tissue biopsy have led to grouping of different forms of vasculitis into 'small-vessel', 'medium-vessel' and 'large-vessel' vasculitis, but some of these descriptions are not disease-specific. In this chapter we will discuss the different forms of vasculitis, their diagnosis and management.

6.2　Diagnosis

The symptoms of vasculitis often depend on the organ involved, e.g. skin, lung or kidneys. There are also some shared common features across different forms of vasculitis, which are discussed below.

6.2.1 Common features of vasculitis

Rash

Classically the rash of vasculitis is a purpuric and non-blanching rash. It can appear very rapidly and is a warning feature of active inflammation. The most common areas where it appears include the lower legs or buttock region, e.g. in Henoch–Schönlein purpura, which is most common in children. In other cases, patients may have changes at the nails, including nailfold infarcts with nail discolouration. The aetiopathogenesis of many of these changes is thought to be immune complex-mediated.

Fatigue

Unexplained fatigue with general malaise is a recognised feature of vasculitis. Since vasculitis is a rare diagnosis in the general population, it is important to investigate for and exclude other conditions causing fatigue which require specific treatment, e.g. anaemia, malignancy and infectious causes.

Systemic symptoms

Fevers, weight loss and night sweats, traditionally known as the 'B' symptoms, are known features of vasculitis. However, several of these symptoms can also overlap with other underlying conditions, e.g. malignancies such as lymphoma. Therefore, in the work-up of cases of vasculitis, general investigations are often performed to confirm the diagnosis; this also includes scans such as CT scans to exclude malignancies such as lymphomas and lymph node or other tissue biopsies of the affected organ.

Neurological

Vasculitis can result in a broad range of neurological features, including an ascending neuropathy which can often cause pain, altered sensation and/or paraesthesia in the affected area, e.g. both feet, legs or arms. Infiltration of nerve tissue with inflammatory cells and blood vessel inflammation are often observed on tissue biopsy of affected nerves; for example, a mononeuritis multiplex is a recognised feature of vasculitis. In large vessel vasculitis, e.g. giant cell arteritis (GCA), patients can present with headache (inflammation of temporal arteries), often unilateral, visual disturbance and even stroke (due to involvement of intracerebral blood vessels).

Respiratory

Lung involvement is often observed in the ANCA-positive vasculitides (see blood tests below). Changes can include presence of pulmonary infiltrates which are visible on CT scan, and also pulmonary fibrosis on HRCT chest scans. Further confirmation of the diagnosis may be required using video-assisted thoracoscopic surgery of affected lung areas.

Renal

Renal involvement is a serious and potentially life-threatening complication of vasculitis. It is important to collect a urine sample in all cases of suspected renal vasculitis and examine the urine for the presence of red cell casts, which typifies an active urinary sediment. The presence of red cell casts and proteinuria are both used to assess disease severity and plan treatment. A renal biopsy is also often performed to classify the changes observed before treatment is initiated.

A number of classification criteria have been developed for the diagnosis of vasculitis, based on the Chapel Hill criteria (Jennette et al., 2013). These include the size of the blood vessels involved (i.e. whether small, medium or large), the presence of immune complexes and the presence of autoantibodies (Table 6.1).

Table 6.1. Types of vasculitis

Type	Name
Large vessel vasculitis	Takayasu's arteritis
	Giant cell arteritis
Medium vessel vasculitis	Polyarteritis nodosa
	Kawasaki's disease

Table 6.1. (Continued)

Type	Name
Small vessel vasculitis	Anti-neutrophil cytoplasmic antibody-associated vasculitis
	Microscopic polyangiitis
	Granulomatous polyangiitis
	Eosinophilic granulomatosis with polyangiitis (EGPA) (Churg–Strauss)
Immune complex small vessel vasculitis	Anti-glomerular basement membrane disease
	Cryoglobulinaemic vasculitis
	IgA vasculitis (Henoch–Schönlein)
	Hypocomplementaemic urticarial vasculitis (anti-C1q)
Variable vessel vasculitis	Behçet's disease
	Cogan's syndrome
Single organ vasculitis	Cutaneous leucocytoclastic angiitis
	Cutaneous arteritis
	Primary central nervous system vasculitis
	Isolated arteritis
Systemic disease-associated vasculitis	Rheumatoid vasculitis
	SLE-related vasculitis
	Sarcoid vasculitis
Other causes	Hepatitis B virus-associated vasculitis
	Hepatitis C virus-associated cryoglobulinaemic vasculitis
	Syphilis-associated aortitis
	Drug-associated immune complex vasculitis
	Drug-associated ANCA-positive vasculitis
	Cancer-associated vasculitis
	Checkpoint inhibitor-related vasculitis

6.2.2 Blood tests

Blood tests which should be performed for vasculitis include the following:

- ESR and CRP: these markers of inflammation are often elevated at presentation. With treatment they can also be used to track disease activity and are often suppressed in response to immunomodulatory treatment.
- ANCA: the anti-neutrophil cytoplasmic antibodies are a very useful test in stratifying the type of vasculitis involved. The antibodies are raised against antigens in the cytoplasm of neutrophil granulocytes. The c-ANCA antigen is specifically proteinase 3 (PR3). Antigens for p-ANCA include myeloperoxidase (MPO) and bacterial permeability increasing factor. Other antigens for c- and p-ANCA are increasingly recognised, but most clinical laboratory enzyme-linked immunosorbent assay (ELISA) tests are specific for PR3 and MPO. Presence of PR3 and MPO antibodies is very helpful in the diagnosis of ANCA-positive vasculitis and in determining treatment strategies.
- ANA: the antinuclear antibody is an antibody targeted to nuclear components of the cell. Although fairly non-specific, the antibody can be a useful indicator of an underlying autoimmune process.
- Complement levels: the complement cascade is part of the immune system that allows antibodies and phagocytic cells to clear microbes and damaged cells from an organism. In autoimmune-mediated vasculitis, instead of phagocytosing microbial pathogens, the complement cascade enhances the ability of autoantibodies and phagocytic cells to clear damaged cells. In active vasculitis, complement C3 and C4 levels are often reduced due to active clearance by antibodies and macrophages, e.g. lupus nephritis. As treatment is initiated and a patient responds to immunomodulatory therapy, the complement C3 and C4 levels may return to the normal range.

6.2.3 Imaging

Modern imaging techniques are very helpful in the diagnosis and monitoring of vasculitis. Techniques such as CT and MRI can be used to identify specific changes, e.g. pulmonary lesions for CT. MRI and CT angiography are useful in identifying the level of vascular involvement. In some specific conditions such as GCA,

Table 6.2. Imaging techniques used in vasculitis

Imaging techniques used in vasculitis	Organ imaged	Contrast used
Ultrasound scan	Temporal arteries	No
Positron emission tomography (PET)	Whole body scan	Yes
Computerised tomography (CT)	Whole body or focused region	Yes
Magnetic resonance imaging (MRI)	Whole body or focused region	No

duplex ultrasonography has very high resolution in diagnosing classical changes such as the 'halo' sign. Duplex ultrasonography in GCA can also have utility in identifying sites for tissue biopsy; these can sometimes be difficult to identify without imaging due to the presence of skip lesions. PET scans can also be used in GCA to detect the level of vascular involvement in larger blood vessels, e.g. aorta and subclavian vessels. Examples of modern imaging techniques used to aid the diagnosis of vasculitis are shown in *Table 6.2*; an example of a PET scan is shown in *Figure 6.1*.

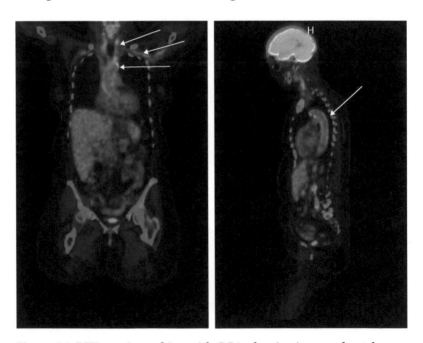

Figure 6.1. PET scan in a subject with GCA, showing increased uptake in the aorta, subclavian and carotid vessels, consistent with a diagnosis of large vessel vasculitis

6.2.4 Biopsy

In many cases of vasculitis, a tissue biopsy is highly desirable. It is helpful not only in confirming the diagnosis, but also in ensuring that there are no other changes, such as cancer, atherosclerosis or infection. A positive biopsy that confirms vasculitic changes is also helpful in justifying strong immunomodulatory medication for a significant period of time.

One of the commonest forms of vasculitis, in which a biopsy is often a critical part of confirming the diagnosis, is giant cell arteritis (GCA). The presenting clinical features of GCA are summarised in *Figure 6.2*. It is usually recommended, if there is a high index of

Management of suspected giant cell arteritis (GCA)

Mandatory criteria
① Age >50; ② CRP >10; ③ New and abrupt onset headache

Plus one or more of:
- Jaw and/or tongue claudication
- New onset visual defect
- Temporal artery abnormalities
- Preceding polymyalgia rheumatica (PMR) symptoms

Immediate investigations
- Serology: FBC, U&E, ESR, CRP, LFT, bone profile + vitamin D
- Urine dip:
  + blood → red cell casts
  + protein → urine protein: CR
  + leucocytes/nitrites → MCS
- CXR
- USS temporal arteries and temporal artery biopsy (urgent)

If high clinical suspicion for GCA

Immediate start of steroid
- GCA without visual compromise: prednisolone 40–60mg daily until resolution of symptom and improvement in inflammatory markers
- GCA with evolving visual loss and/or amaurosis fugax: consider IV methylprednisolone 500–1000mg daily for 3 days before switching to oral steroid following senior clinician or Rheumatology review
- GCA with established visual loss: prednisolone 60mg or 1mg/kg daily

Bone protection: alendronic acid + Adcal D3
Gastrointestinal protection

Figure 6.2. Pathway for assessment of suspected GCA

suspicion for GCA, that patients undergo ultrasound of the temporal arteries to assess for the presence of the 'halo' sign and also to assist in marking the site for temporal artery biopsy. If GCA is suspected, then immediate high dose corticosteroid therapy is recommended, as summarised in *Figure 6.2*.

6.3 Causes

Vasculitis covers a very wide spectrum of conditions, summarised in *Table 6.1*. There are certain environmental factors which are known to be associated with the development of vasculitis, e.g. infections including hepatitis B, C and syphilis (see *Figure 6.3*). Certain drugs are also associated with the development of vasculitis, including antibiotics such as cephalosporins, penicillins and the newly developed and licensed checkpoint inhibitors for the treatment of a wide range of cancers. A summary of factors known to contribute to the development of vasculitis is shown in *Figure 6.3*.

6.4 Management

Initial education about the condition is important, as in general, vasculitis is rare and patients may not know much about the wide range of conditions that include vasculitis. Charities including Versus Arthritis and Vasculitis UK have websites for patients and carers providing up-to-date information (www.versusarthritis.org/; www.vasculitis.org.uk).

With respect to pharmacological therapy, treatment is focused on induction treatment, followed by maintenance therapy. At the induction phase, the aim is to achieve remission of the disease. After induction treatment, therapy then moves into the maintenance phase in order to prevent the development of relapses.

6.4.1 Induction phase

Treatment in the induction phase has dramatically improved in the last few decades. Initially it is aimed at controlling the acute

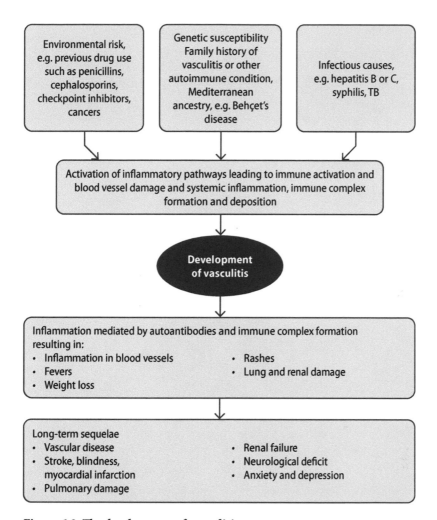

Figure 6.3. The development of vasculitis

inflammatory response to salvage function, depending on the organ involved, e.g. sight in GCA or renal function in renal vasculitis. Induction treatment often includes high dose corticosteroids, e.g. pulsed IV methylprednisolone such as 1g per day for 3 days, in addition to treatment with pulsed cyclophosphamide. In more recent years, introduction of the B-cell depleting antibody rituximab has also significantly improved outcomes for vasculitis. Protocols exist based on large multicentre studies; for example the Eurolupus regime for cyclophosphamide (Harper *et al.*, 2012) includes pulsed or oral cyclophosphamide over a period of up to 3–6 months.

Table 6.3. Disease-modifying therapies used for the management of vasculitis

Drug	Formulation and dose	Mechanism of action	Usual level of therapy (NICE guidelines)	Screening	Monitoring
Corticosteroids, e.g. prednisolone, methylprednisolone	PO/IM/IV	Works through multiple pathways including increased transcription of anti-inflammatory genes	Induction	Monitor for diabetes, hypertension	FBC, U+Es, LFTs
Cyclophosphamide	PO/IV	Cytotoxic agent	Induction	Hepatitis B & C, HIV, TB	FBC, U+Es, LFTs
Rituximab (Mabthera, Truxima biosimilar)	IV 1g 2 weeks apart then after 6 months	Monoclonal antibody to CD20	Induction	Hepatitis B & C, HIV, TB B-cell subsets	FBC, U+Es, LFTs
Tocilizumab (Actemra)	IV/SC every 4 weeks	Monoclonal antibody to IL-6 receptor	Induction	Hepatitis B & C, HIV, TB	FBC, U+Es, LFTs, lipids
Sarilumab (Kevzara)	200mg SC every 2 weeks	Monoclonal antibody to IL-6 receptor	Induction	Hepatitis B & C, HIV, TB	FBC, U+Es, LFTs, lipids
IV immunoglobulin	Total dose 2g/kg	Inhibition of autoantibody activity, T cells, dendritic cells, complement	Induction	Baseline levels of immunoglobulins	FBC, U+Es, LFTs
Methotrexate	PO/SC Typically 15–25mg weekly	Inhibition of purine synthesis	Maintenance	Hepatitis B & C, HIV	FBC, U+Es, LFTs
Leflunomide	PO Typically 20mg daily after loading dose	Inhibition of pyrimidine synthesis	Maintenance	Hepatitis B & C, HIV	FBC, U+Es, LFTs
Azathioprine	PO Typically 50–150mg daily in divided doses	Inhibition of purine synthesis	Maintenance	Hepatitis B & C, HIV	FBC, U+Es, LFTs
Hydroxychloroquine	PO Up to 400mg daily in divided doses	Inhibitor of expression of TNF and other cytokines	Maintenance	Hepatitis B & C, HIV	FBC, U+Es, LFTs
Mycophenolate mofetil	PO Up to 1.5g bd, total daily dose 3g in divided doses	Inhibits T and B cell proliferation	Maintenance	Hepatitis B & C, HIV	FBC, U+Es, LFTs

In severe cases, subjects may require plasma exchange, dialysis or even renal transplant.

Since cyclophosphamide is a cytotoxic drug, patients do require informed consent for its use. Patients need to be warned of side-effects including hair loss, nausea, vomiting, impaired fertility and infection risk. For female patients of child-bearing age, if they are considering pregnancy in the future after several cycles of cyclophosphamide therapy, they may require referral to a fertility clinic before treatment, for egg storage. An alternative treatment to cyclophosphamide, namely rituximab, may have fewer side-effects in fertility and may be more appropriate in some cases where treatment is required in women of child-bearing age.

6.4.2 Maintenance phase

Once organ function has been maintained, maintenance therapy for vasculitis may be required to maintain disease remission using DMARDs, including mycophenolate mofetil, azathioprine and methotrexate. Such treatments may need to be continued for several years to maintain disease remission and to prevent the development of relapses. Relapses can often require further treatment with therapies such as pulsed corticosteroid, cyclophosphamide or rituximab. A summary of the treatments used for the management of vasculitis is shown in *Table 6.3*.

6.5 Cases

The following cases are based on real patients and are presented to help you consider how you would manage the scenarios.

Case history 6.1

A 64-year-old British Indian lady presented to A&E with a 4-month history of 9kg weight loss, night sweats, fevers and weakness around her shoulder girdle. In the last few weeks she had also developed a left-sided headache and blurred vision. She had travelled to India approximately 6 months previously but had no other significant travel history. She was admitted under the infectious diseases team for further investigations.

She underwent investigations for TB, hepatitis A, B and C, HIV, syphilis and cytomegalovirus, all of which were negative. Her blood results were as follows: Hb 90g/L, white cell count 7.2×10^9/L, platelets 568×10^9, ESR 110mm/hr, CRP 98g/L, ALT 88, estimated glomerular filtration rate (eGFR) 54. Her chest radiograph was normal. She has a CT chest, abdomen and pelvis which showed mild emphysema but no other changes.

What would be the next investigation(s) of choice?

- Lymph node biopsy
- HRCT chest
- PET scan
- US temporal arteries
- White cell scan

The differential diagnosis includes vasculitis, with the most likely cause being GCA, in view of the headache, visual changes and systemic symptoms. The patient required an US scan of the temporal arteries, which confirmed the presence of the 'halo' sign. She also had a PET scan to exclude malignancy and investigate the extent of the vasculitis. The PET scan showed the presence of increased tracer uptake in the ascending aorta and subclavian vessels.

The patient was started on pulsed IV methylprednisolone 500mg per day in three daily doses, followed by oral prednisolone 60mg daily. After 3 days, her ESR had dropped to 56mm/hr and her CRP was down to 34g/L.

What other treatment should be initiated?

- A proton pump inhibitor
- Calcichew D3
- Alendronic acid
- Aspirin
- Methotrexate

In the acute management of GCA, patients will require gastroprotection to cover treatment with high dose corticosteroids. Bone protection is also recommended to prevent the development of osteopenia and subsequent fractures, and is often initiated with a combination of calcium and vitamin D supplements, and bisphosphonates if there are no contraindications. Long-term DMARD therapy is not usually commenced early in diagnosis; rather it is considered if dose reduction with steroid is not possible and steroid-sparing agents are required.

Case history 6.2

A 47-year-old man presented to his GP surgery with a 2-week history of haemoptysis. He initially coughed up blood on one occasion, but this was now a daily occurrence. He also experienced shortness of breath. He was referred to the medical team in the hospital for further assessment. On examination, he was found to have saturations of 92% on room air. He reported that he had also noted a few episodes of blood in his urine. He was admitted for further tests.

He had a chest radiograph which showed bilateral pulmonary infiltrates. He also had evidence of urinary casts on urinalysis. His blood results were as below:

Hb 105g/L, total white cell count 11.1×10^9, neutrophils 2.0×10^9, eosinophils 1.1×10^9, ESR 55mm/hr, CRP 68g/L.

What is the most likely diagnosis?

- Tuberculosis
- Carcinoma of the lung
- *Mycoplasma* pneumonia
- Eosinophilic granulomatosis with polyangiitis (EGPA)
- Interstitial lung disease

The most likely diagnosis is eosinophilic granulomatosis with polyangiitis (EGPA). The patient had a peripheral blood eosinophilia, haemoptysis, pulmonary infiltrates and an active urinary sediment. Lung biopsy confirmed vasculitis. He was treated with 6 pulses of IV cyclophosphamide induction treatment, followed by maintenance therapy with oral azathioprine. He remains in remission and has not had any flare-ups of his vasculitis. His eosinophil count and renal function have returned to normal.

Case history 6.3

A 32-year-old woman presented to A&E with pain and swelling in her left ankle. She initially developed pain followed by swelling in the ankle and in the last few days had also noticed a rash developing over her shin (see image below). Initially the rash was painless, but she had found it to be increasingly itchy. She had also noticed numbness in her feet. Due to the severity of the skin changes, she went on to have a skin biopsy.

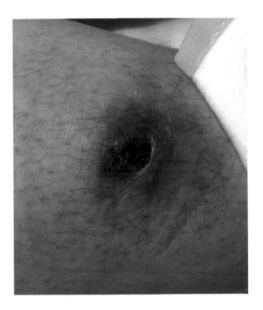

What is the most likely diagnosis?

- Cutaneous vasculitis with neurological involvement
- Diabetic ulcer
- Erythema nodosum
- Cellulitis
- Wegener's granulomatosis

The skin biopsy confirmed active vasculitis, with infiltration of B cells and leucocytoclastic changes. The patient also has nerve conduction studies which showed a small fibre peripheral neuropathy. She agreed to treatment with IV pulsed methylprednisolone 500mg over 3 days. After this treatment she noticed a significant clinical improvement of the numbness in her feet. She was then started on mycophenolate mofetil 500mg three times daily. After 6 weeks her rash had improved significantly. She continued with mycophenolate mofetil and was reviewed regularly in clinic every three months. Twelve months after her initial presentation, she was reviewed in the Rheumatology clinic. Her rash had resolved and she had no further neurological symptoms. She reported to the Rheumatology team that she planned to start a family and would like some advice for the best disease-modifying treatment to keep her vasculitis under control during conception and pregnancy.

Which disease-modifying drug(s) would it be safe to prescribe in pregnancy?

- Mycophenolate mofetil
- Hydroxychloroquine
- Methotrexate
- Sulfasalazine
- Cyclophosphamide

Hydroxychloroquine and sulfasalazine are considered safe in pregnancy, but other agents including mycophenolate mofetil, methotrexate and cyclophosphamide all have highly teratogenic effects and are not considered to be safe during pregnancy and breastfeeding. The patient decided to switch to hydroxychloroquine and stopped mycophenolate mofetil. Her vasculitis remained quiescent and she went on to have a successful pregnancy with her baby born at term.

Case history 6.4

A 36-year-old plumber came to the ED with an acutely swollen right leg. It had developed over the last few days. He had not had any previous episodes of this kind. Apart from noticing a few mouth ulcers, he has had no other symptoms. He had no other significant past medical history, except an episode of red eye (which he was told was uveitis) in his early twenties. On examination he had three mouth ulcers and was noted to have an ulcer on the penis. Clinically he had a right above-knee deep vein thrombosis which was also confirmed on Doppler US scan.

What is the most likely unifying diagnosis?

- *Neisseria gonorrhoeae* infection
- Syphilis infection
- Behçet's disease
- Lymphoma
- Ankylosing spondylitis

The history and clinical findings are consistent with Behçet's disease, which is a unique form of vasculitis with multisystem involvement and unknown aetiology. There is a typical geographical distribution, in people of Mediterranean and Asian origin, spanning the distance of the Silk Route. Criteria for diagnosis include recurrent oral and genital ulceration, eye lesions (including anterior/posterior uveitis and retinal vasculitis), skin lesions such as erythema nodosum, thromboses and a positive pathergy test. A pathergy test is an exaggerated skin reaction occurring after trauma such as a bump or bruise. A pathergy test is usually performed by applying a sterile needle with multiple pricks to the forearm. After 48 hours, a positive test is interpreted by the presence of a large red bump, pustule or ulceration.

The patient was started on colchicine for his ulcers, which responded well. He was also treated with an oral anticoagulant, rivaroxaban, for 6 months, following which his deep vein thrombosis resolved.

6.6 References

Harper, L., Morgan, M.D., Walsh, M. *et al.* (2012) Pulse versus daily oral cyclophosphamide for induction of remission in ANCA-associated vasculitis: long-term follow-up. *Ann Rheum Dis.*, **71(6):** 955–60.

Hellmich, B., Agueda, A., Monti, S. *et al.* (2020) 2018 Update of the EULAR recommendations for the management of large vessel vasculitis. *Ann Rheum Dis.*, **79(1):** 19–30.

Jennette, J.C., Falk, R.J., Bacon, P.A. *et al.* (2013) 2012 revised International Chapel Hill Consensus Conference nomenclature of vasculitides. *Arthritis Rheum.*, **65(1):** 1–11.

Wallace, Z.S. and Miloslavsky, E.M. (2020) Management of ANCA associated vasculitis. *BMJ,* **368:**m421.

NICE and BSR guidelines

NICE guidelines for the use of tocilizumab in giant cell arteritis www.nice.org.uk/guidance/ta518

NICE guidelines for the management of ANCA-positive vasculitis with rituximab www.nice.org.uk/Guidance/TA308.

Ntatsaki, E., Carruthers, D., Chakravarty, K. *et al.* (2014) BSR and BHPR guideline for the management of adults with ANCA-associated vasculitis. *Rheumatology,* **53(12):** 2306–9.

Charities providing patient support

www.vasculitis.org.uk/

www.versusarthritis.org

CHAPTER 7

Osteoarthritis

7.1 Introduction

Osteoarthritis (OA) is the most common form of arthritis worldwide, affecting over 8 million people in the UK alone. OA is a heterogeneous condition, which can typically affect different joint regions, including the hands and larger weight-bearing joints such as the knees and hips. Spinal disease is also an important cause of morbidity and time lost to work. OA is a disease of the whole joint and is characterised by changes in the cartilage, bone and synovium. The age of onset is typically >50 years. The female to male ratio is approximately 1.7: 1. In this chapter we will discuss the different forms of OA, their diagnosis and management.

7.2 Diagnosis

The symptoms of OA can depend on the region involved. The most common symptoms include pain in the affected joint on activity, stiffness and impaired function. Traditionally, the early morning stiffness that is associated with inflammatory arthritides such as rheumatoid arthritis and ankylosing spondylitis, which at its worst can last more than 30 minutes and often up to several hours each day, is usually shorter in OA and can last up to 30 minutes. In recent years, it has been proposed that OA can be stratified into distinct forms (see *Table 7.1*), which can assist in developing care pathways for the different types of OA. Distinct OA subtypes are discussed further below.

7.2.1 Subtypes of osteoarthritis

Hand

Hand OA mainly involves the first carpometacarpal (CMC) joint of the thumbs, proximal interphalangeal (PIP) joints and distal interphalangeal (DIP) joints. There is an increased prevalence of this condition in women compared to men. Risk factors include genetic risk, manual jobs and previous injuries to finger joints. Blood tests and radiographs (see *Figure 7.1*) are used to aid the diagnosis. Bony overgrowth and osteophyte formation lead to the development of Heberden's nodes (DIP joints) and Bouchard's nodes (PIP joints). Once nodes develop, they reach a maximum size. During their growth and development, Heberden's and Bouchard's nodes are painful. Once they reach a maximum size, the pain in these regions tends to regress, but the deformities which develop are irreversible (see plain radiographs in *Figure 7.1*).

Large joint

Hip and knee OA are the most prevalent and symptomatic forms of OA. Symptoms include pain focused on the joint, reduced range of movement, locking, giving way and swelling. Swelling of the knee joint usually indicates a flare-up due to the accumulation of synovial fluid, which in some cases is also associated with synovitis. In some cases, people with shoulder, hip, knee or foot OA can also experience referred pain; for example, hip OA can be associated with pain referred to the knee. Plain radiographs are often used to confirm the diagnosis and more pathological changes can also be seen by MRI scan, e.g. synovitis and bone marrow oedema (see *Figure 7.1*). The most common radiographic features are osteophyte formation, sclerosis, joint space narrowing and subchondral cyst formation. In some cases, MRI may also be used to exclude other causes of pain, e.g. meniscal tear or anterior cruciate ligament tear.

Spinal

Spinal OA most commonly affects the cervical region and lumbar area. It is typified by pain in those regions and reduced range of movement; for example, inability to turn the spine to the side or bend forwards. If there is associated disc herniation, there can be impingement of nerve roots and sciatic symptoms, often called 'sciatica'. Some people can develop 'bridging osteophytes' between

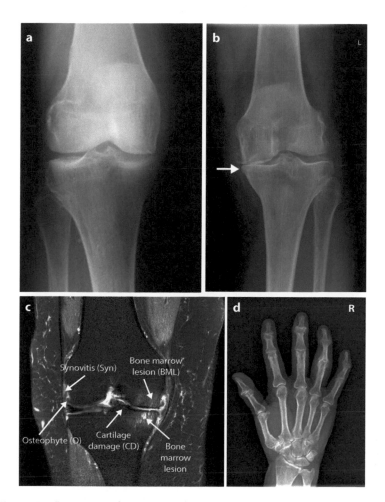

Figure 7.1. Imaging techniques used in osteoarthritis
(a) Plain radiograph of normal knee; (b) plain radiograph of advanced
OA, showing joint space narrowing of the medial compartment of the knee
(arrow), sclerosis of the bone and a subchondral cyst; (c) MRI scan of knee
shows several characteristic changes of OA, including cartilage damage and
osteophyte formation. Other changes which are appreciated on MRI are
usually not visible on plain radiography, including synovitis and bone marrow
lesions (BMLs). BMLs are known to correlate with pain in OA; (d) Typical
radiographic changes in hand OA, showing involvement of the DIP, PIP and
1st CMC joints of the hand.

vertebrae, which can result in pain and restricted movement. Others
may develop osteoarthritic changes at the facet joint, which can be
detected radiographically.

Table 7.1. Subtypes of osteoarthritis

Subgroups of OA based on risk factors	Aetiology	Joint affected
Bone and cartilage	The primary changes observed are damage to cartilage and bone Cartilage degradation and bone marrow lesions are seen	Foot, hand, hip, knee, shoulder
Chronic pain	The predominant symptom is high reporting of pain Some people have referred pain and others have features of pain sensitisation Radiographic damage is minimal in some cases and advanced in others	Knee, hip, hand, spine
Inflammatory	Typified by erosions and active synovitis	Erosive hand osteoarthritis Knee and hip inflammatory OA
Metabolic syndrome	Associated with diabetes mellitus, obesity, hypertension, gout, elevated urate levels	Foot, hand, hip, knee
Perimenopausal	Often occurs in women at the time of menopause or during chemotherapy, e.g. anti-oestrogens for breast cancer	Hand most common Also occurs in hip, knee, spine
Post-traumatic OA	Mechanical overload on affected joints	Foot, hip, knee, shoulder

7.2.2 Blood tests

Tests which should be performed to confirm the diagnosis of OA include the following:

- ESR and CRP: these markers of inflammation are expected to be in the normal range in OA (see *Appendix* for further details)
- ANA, RhF and anti-CCP antibodies: these are often checked to exclude any evidence of inflammatory arthritis

- It should be noted that OA can coexist with other forms of arthritis, including gout, CPPD, RA and PsA. In some forms of arthritis, e.g. gout, the weakness in joint tissue created by the damaged joint due to OA often leads to a cycle of accumulation of crystals, which can cause further damage and inflammation in the joint, leading to pain and swelling.

7.2.3 Imaging

Imaging techniques are very helpful in the diagnosis and management of OA. The most commonly used tool in the clinic is plain radiography. In some cases, ultrasound may be used, e.g. to detect the level of synovitis if an inflammatory subtype of OA is suspected. In other cases, MRI may be used to assist in establishing if there is a traumatic basis to the OA, e.g. meniscal tear or anterior cruciate ligament tear of the knee. Examples of imaging changes are shown in *Figure 7.1*.

7.3 Causes

As summarised in *Table 7.1*, OA can be due to a number of risk factors, which range from trauma to obesity, metabolic syndrome and inflammatory subtypes. The causes of OA are shown in *Figure 7.2*. One of the strongest risk factors for OA is obesity. There are also certain genetic conditions which are associated with an increased risk of development of OA, including type II collagen mutations: Stickler's syndrome.

7.4 Management

The management of OA is often multidisciplinary. Since it is a chronic condition, with the development of symptoms over a long period of time, it is important to tailor management at the level of the patient's symptoms. The NICE guidelines for OA recommend a multidisciplinary approach to care (www.nice.org.uk/Guidance/CG177), summarised in *Table 7.2*.

125

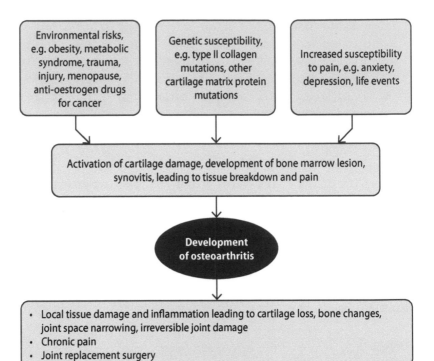

Figure 7.2. The development of osteoarthritis

Table 7.2. NICE guidelines for the management of osteoarthritis

Type of management	Intervention
Non-pharmacological	Supports and braces
	Shock-absorbing shoes or insoles
	TENS machine
	Manual therapy (manipulation and stretching)
Lifestyle interventions	Education and advice
	Strengthening exercises, physiotherapy
	Aerobic fitness training
	Weight loss if overweight/obese
Pharmacological management	NSAIDs, opioids, capsaicin, steroid injections
Surgery	Autologous chondrocyte implantation
	Joint replacement surgery

Abbreviation: TENS, transcutaneous electrical nerve stimulation.

Treatments can be divided into non-pharmacological and pharmacological, summarised below.

7.4.1 Non-pharmacological

Non-pharmacological therapies should always be used as a first-line treatment.

Education

Patient education is essential to successful outcomes. It is important to provide reassurance to the patient about their diagnosis. Seek to address any fears and anxieties the patient may have. Work on patient-centred goals, taking into account patient expectations and their understanding of their condition. Try to encourage normal activities and self-management strategies. Explore other lifestyle factors such as poor sleep, stress, anxiety, depression, nutrition and poor self-efficacy, which can also determine outcome.

Provide information on sources of advice and support, such as:
- Versus Arthritis (www.versusarthritis.org), a national charity which provides information and support for people with arthritis, including information leaflets on OA, hip pain and OA of the knee, covering different joint involvement, self-management strategies, medical and surgical treatments.
- Arthritis and Musculoskeletal Alliance (ARMA; arma.uk.net), a national action network aiming to improve standards of care for people in the UK with arthritis and other musculoskeletal disorders by encouraging cooperation between charities and professional organisations.
- The NHS information leaflet on osteoarthritis (www.nhs.uk/conditions/osteoarthritis).

Physiotherapy

It is important to maintain strength and function by learning and participating in regular exercise. Many tools are now freely available online, including the ESCAPE-pain website tools with free videos (https://escape-pain.org/external-exercise-videos). The exercise regime is based on activities to strengthen and tone the muscles, tendons and ligaments of the lower limb to provide increased power and stability, including the quadriceps/hamstring muscle groups and also strengthening muscles around the hips and feet. Typical exercises include sit to stand exercises, heel slides, knee wedge exercises, squats, hamstring stretch, standing on one leg, isometric squats and using the exercise bike.

Exercise

Exercise is effective in reducing pain and improving physical function in knee OA (Fransen *et al.*, 2015; Zhang *et al.*, 2010). Exercise programmes should focus on improving quadriceps and hamstring strength, as patients often have reduced muscle strength due to reduced physical activity and pain inhibition. These types of exercises can reduce joint loading. Aerobic exercise should also be included as it aims to increase heart rate and oxygen uptake. It is known that people with OA are much more likely to also have hypertension, obesity and cardiovascular disease, often due to these shared risk factors. Increasing aerobic exercise improves not only cardiac and lung function, but also blood flow and metabolic activity and turnover in the muscles, tendons and tissue in joint structures. Increased aerobic activity can be achieved by swimming, cycling or running. The optimal exercise 'dose' has not been substantiated but evidence suggests programmes should be supervised, be performed 2–3 times per week and consist of at least 12 sessions. Exercise recommendations should be taken into account regarding patient preference, access and affordability (Kolasinski *et al.*, 2020). It is important that exercise doesn't cause symptoms to flare up, although small flare-ups that settle within 24 hours are acceptable. In some patients, activity modification may be indicated, for example walking rather than running, or doing aquatic exercises. Mind and body exercises have been recommended by the ACR/AF 2019 and OARSI guidelines (Bannuru *et al.*, 2019).

Physical supports

Several physical devices can be used to support joints, e.g. taping of the hands, bracing of the thumb and knee, and insoles in the feet (see *Figure 7.3*). They not only provide support but may also improve stability and balance, e.g. insoles. Further advice on use of braces and taping can be accessed from the Versus Arthritis website (www.versusarthritis.org/media/1259/osteoarthritis-of-the-knee-information-booklet.pdf).

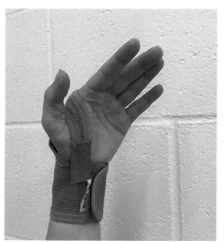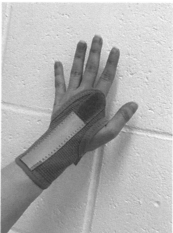

Figure 7.3. Wrist and thumb brace for CMC osteoarthritis

Acupuncture

The efficacy of acupuncture remains controversial and it has not been recommended by either the NICE 2019 or the OARSI guidelines. The ACR/AF guidelines recommend traditional Chinese acupuncture for patients with chronic moderate to severe pain who would be candidates for total knee arthroplasty but either do not want it or have contraindications (Kolasinski *et al.*, 2020).

7.4.2 Pharmacological

Drug treatment is largely focused on pain management (*Table 7.3*). These include paracetamol, NSAIDs and opioids. NICE recommendations suggest that the lowest dose of analgesic should be prescribed for the shortest duration of time, with paracetamol recommended as first line. NSAIDs have proven efficacy in OA, and a wide variety of NSAIDs, including non-COX selective and COX-II selective NSAIDs can be prescribed. NSAIDs may be associated with significant side-effects, including GI upset such as gastritis and peptic ulcer disease. If mild, such symptoms can be controlled with PPIs such as omeprazole or lansoprazole. Other side-effects which require monitoring include renal function and monitoring of respiratory symptoms, e.g asthma. If NSAIDs are associated with significant side-effects, or there is ongoing lack of analgesic effect, opioids may be used. The most commonly prescribed opioid analgesics for OA include codeine-based analgesics.

CHAPTER 7: OSTEOARTHRITIS

Table 7.3. Pharmacological management of osteoarthritis

Drug	Formulation and dose	Mechanism of action	Usual level of therapy (NICE guidelines)	Screening	Monitoring
NSAIDs	PO/SC Typically ibuprofen 400mg 3 times daily in divided doses	Inhibition of cyclooxygenase I and II pathways	1st line	Check for previous GI peptic ulcer disease, renal function, asthma	FBC, U+Es, LFTs
Opioids	PO Typically e.g. codeine and paracetamol 15/500 up to 8 tablets daily	Inhibition of opioid-mediated pain pathways	1st line	No previous side-effects, respiratory problems, constipation	FBC, U+Es, LFTs
Capsaicin	Topical 0.025–0.05 micrograms	Modulates TRPV channels around skin and joint	1st line	Check for any skin rashes where the cream is applied and avoid open wounds	Check for any skin rashes
Corticosteroids, e.g. Depo-Medrone	Intra-articular	Works through multiple pathways including increased transcription of anti-inflammatory genes	1st line	Monitor for diabetes, hypertension, check for any skin changes or infection	Monitor for joint flare or infection
Hyaluronic acid	Intra-articular	Improved lubrication of the joint, allowing easier movement	2nd line	Check for any skin changes or infection	Monitor for joint flare or infection

Abbreviation: TRPV, transient receptor potential vanilloid.

130

Unfortunately, there are currently no proven disease-modifying therapies which are licensed for the management of OA that delay progression of the disease. Several clinical trials have been carried out, including hydroxychloroquine for hand OA and methotrexate for knee OA. Problems with some of the trials have included inadequate subtyping of different forms of OA, e.g. inflammatory versus primarily cartilage and bone changes, but this is an area of active research. Further trials are currently underway, including biologic treatments for pain management in OA, e.g. anti-nerve growth factor antibodies.

Some patients use nutraceutical drugs such as glucosamine and chondroitin sulphate, which are advertised widely to alleviate pain and improve function. Currently such drugs are not recommended by NICE, since they do not appear to have significantly increased efficacy over NSAIDs over a sustained period of time.

7.5 Cases

The following cases are based on real patients and are presented to help you consider how you would manage the scenarios.

Case history 7.1

A 75-year-old man presents with acute pain and swelling of his right knee. On examination there is reduced range of movement with a positive patellar tap. He is overweight. There is no history of previous trauma, joint pain or swelling.

What is the single most important investigation to perform?

- Aspiration of knee joint synovial fluid
- Serum urate
- Blood cultures
- CRP measurement
- Serum RhF

The patient requires aspiration of the joint fluid in order to establish the diagnosis. The knee aspirate does not show any crystals or inflammatory cells and the Gram stain is negative. A plain radiograph of the knee shows joint space narrowing consistent with OA. The patient is in pain. His other medications include amlodipine for hypertension.

What would be the first treatment of choice for pain control?

- Oral corticosteroids
- Ibuprofen
- Codeine phosphate
- Morphine sulphate
- Amitriptyline

Oral NSAIDs are the first treatment of choice during an acute flare of OA, as in this case. If the patient has side-effects on NSAIDs, an alternative can be considered such as codeine phosphate. The patient improved with ibuprofen and physiotherapy and was discharged home. If the patient stops responding to NSAIDs and physiotherapy, corticosteroid injections could be considered in future management. Corticosteroids are recommended by NICE in cases where subjects have not responded fully to treatment with NSAIDs, other analgesics such as opioids, or physiotherapy. However, injections are usually limited to 3 injections for any joint in a lifetime.

Case history 7.2

A 65-year-old retired plumber came to see his GP. He has had pain in his right hip for the last 3 months. The pain is worse when he has been standing for long periods or when he stands up from a seated position. There is no night pain. He has taken paracetamol and ibuprofen 400mg three times daily but still has ongoing pain. The GP arranges a plain radiograph of the hips and pelvis. The X-ray confirms that the patient has moderately severe OA of the right hip, with joint space narrowing and osteophytes.

What does the GP do next?

- Switches the patient to topical NSAIDs
- Switches to naproxen 500mg bd and paracetamol
- Refers the patient for physiotherapy
- Arranges a corticosteroid injection into the hip under ultrasound guidance
- Refers the patient for joint replacement surgery

All the options given are plausible. A multidisciplinary approach is required, including adequate pain control, physiotherapy and potentially steroid injection. All these options are usually explored first before the patient is referred for joint replacement surgery.

Case history 7.3

A 54-year-old woman is referred to the hand clinic. She has severe pain in her thumbs. The pain has been worsening for the last 6 months. On questioning, she tells the doctor in the hand clinic that she has recently gone through the menopause and has had chemotherapy for breast cancer.

What treatment is the woman likely to have had for breast cancer which has contributed to her hand pain?

- Herceptin
- Morphine sulphate
- Mastectomy
- Radiotherapy
- Letrozole

Some forms of chemotherapy, e.g. letrozole, can contribute to exacerbated symptoms of joint pain. Letrozole lowers the levels of oestrogen in the body and is often used for up to 5 years for the management of breast cancer. Drugs such as letrozole can exacerbate OA symptoms. The patient was also going through the menopause, which could have worsened her symptoms further. The patient could not stop the letrozole, so she was offered corticosteroid injections into both first CMC joints, which improved her symptoms. She was also referred to hand therapy for hand exercises and taping, which helped to control her symptoms significantly.

7.6 References

Bannuru, R.R., Osani, M.C., Vaysbrot, E.E. *et al.* (2019) OARSI guidelines for the non-surgical management of knee, hip and polyarticular osteoarthritis. *Osteoarthritis Cartilage*, **27(11)**: 1578–1589.

Fernandes, L., Hagen, K.B., Bijlsma, J.W. *et al.* (2013) EULAR recommendations for the non-pharmacological core management of hip and knee osteoarthritis. *Ann Rheum Dis.*, **72(7)**: 1125–1135.

Fransen, M., McConnell, S., Harmer, A.R. *et al.* (2015) Exercise for osteoarthritis of the knee: a Cochrane systematic review. *Br J Sports Med.*, **49(24)**: 1554–1557.

Kloppenburg, M., Kroon, F.P., Blanco, F.J. *et al.* (2019) 2018 update of the EULAR recommendations for the management of hand osteoarthritis. *Ann Rheum Dis.*, **78(1)**: 16–24.

Kolasinski, S.L., Neogi, T., Hochberg, M.C. *et al.* (2020) 2019 American College of Rheumatology/Arthritis Foundation guideline for the management of osteoarthritis of the hand, hip, and knee. *Arthritis Care Res.*, **72(2)**: 149–162.

NICE guidelines and useful websites

NICE guidelines for the management of osteoarthritis:
www.nice.org.uk/Guidance/CG177

NHS patient information for osteoarthritis:
www.nhs.uk/conditions/osteoarthritis/

Zhang, W., Doherty, M., Peat, G. *et al.* (2010) EULAR evidence-based recommendations for the diagnosis of knee osteoarthritis. *Ann Rheum Dis.*, **69(3)**: 483–489.

Versus Arthritis:
www.versusarthritis.org/about-arthritis/conditions/osteoarthritis/

www.versusarthritis.org/media/1259/osteoarthritis-of-the-knee-information-booklet.pdf

www.csp.org.uk/conditions/managing-pain-home/managing-your-knee-pain

CHAPTER 8

Osteoporosis

8.1 Introduction

Osteoporosis is a condition primarily affecting the bone. It is a condition that is characterised by the loss of bone mass which occurs at an accelerated rate compared with normal physiological bone loss. Osteoporosis is a prevalent condition in the UK, affecting more than 3 million people. The risk of osteoporosis increases with age, with women being 4 times more likely than men to develop it. Women are more likely to develop osteoporosis because bone loss becomes more rapid after the menopause, when ovarian production of oestrogen falls. Men also reach higher peak bone mass than women before bone loss begins, and therefore need to lose much greater bone mass before they reach levels consistent with osteoporosis.

8.2 Diagnosis

Osteoporosis is often not associated with specific symptoms such as pain or stiffness in the affected region. The first sign that osteoporosis may exist in a patient could be that they present with a fracture. However, there are several risk factors which can be identified to discuss with patients their likelihood of developing a fracture and how this could be prevented.

Risk factors for osteoporosis include the following:
- Increasing age (> age 60)
- Female gender

- Family history in first-degree relative
- Body mass index (BMI) of ≤19kg/m²
- Previous endocrine or metabolic disorder, e.g. thyroid disease, Cushing's syndrome, hyperparathyroidism, pituitary disorders
- Excessive alcohol intake or smoking
- Long-term use of certain medications, e.g. corticosteroids for arthritis or asthma
- Rheumatoid arthritis
- Drugs used for treatment of cancer, e.g. breast cancer in women and prostate cancer in men
- Early menopause (< age 45)
- Hysterectomy
- Eating disorders, e.g. anorexia or bulimia
- Conditions leading to malabsorption, e.g. Crohn's disease, coeliac disease
- Prolonged periods of immobility.

A number of investigations can be performed to assist in the diagnosis of osteoporosis, which can help inform patients of their risk of developing fractures and plan treatment for prevention of fractures.

8.2.1 DEXA scanning

Dual energy X-ray absorptiometry (DEXA) is a method of measuring bone density using spectral imaging. Two X-ray beams which have different energy levels are aimed at a specific region of bone, e.g. vertebral spine or hip. The absorption by the soft tissue is subtracted out and the bone mineral density (BMD) can be determined from the absorption of each beam by bone.

A number of defined threshold values have been set by the World Health Organization (WHO) for osteopenia (which is low bone density preceding osteoporosis) and osteoporosis. Values for osteopenia and osteoporosis are summarised in *Table 8.1*. The reference measurement is derived from bone density measurements in a population of healthy young adults, called a T-score. Osteoporosis is diagnosed when the BMD is ≥2.5 standard deviations below the reference measurement. Many DEXA reports also provide the Z-score, which is a comparison of a person's bone density with that of an average person of the same age and gender.

Table 8.1. Summary of ranges for BMD in diagnosing osteoporosis

Status	Hip BMD
Normal	T-score of –1 or above
Osteopenia	T-score between –1 and –2.5
Osteoporosis	T-score of –2.5 or lower
Severe osteoporosis	T-score of –2.5 or lower, and presence of at least one fragility fracture

8.2.2 Plain spine X-ray

Sometimes loss of height and subsequent back pain can be the first symptoms of vertebral fractures induced by osteoporosis. The severity of vertebral fractures can be assessed using a semi-quantitative method. The severity of the fracture is assessed by measuring the extent of vertebral height reduction, by changes in bone morphology and by evaluating the changes in deformities which are fracture- and non-fracture-related. Each vertebra can be assigned grades based on the degree of height reduction. *Figure 8.1* shows radiographic features of peri-articular osteopenia in a patient with inflammatory arthritis.

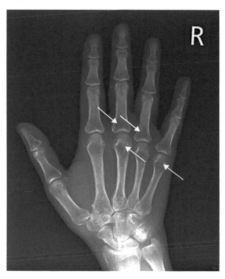

Figure 8.1. Periarticular osteopenia in a patient with inflammatory arthritis
Arrows mark areas of osteopenia.

Since only 30% of vertebral fractures present clinically, thoracic and lumbar spine radiographs can be useful to diagnose subclinical vertebral fractures, and the changes observed can assist in making the diagnosis of osteoporosis. Spinal radiographs can also assist in categorising the severity of vertebral fractures and assessing whether multiple fractures are present at several levels. *Figure 8.2* shows the Genant classification for vertebral fractures, which classifies the degree of fracture severity. In patients >75 years, when DEXA scanning is less sensitive and specific, spinal radiographs can be a useful way of diagnosing osteoporosis if vertebral fractures are found to be present.

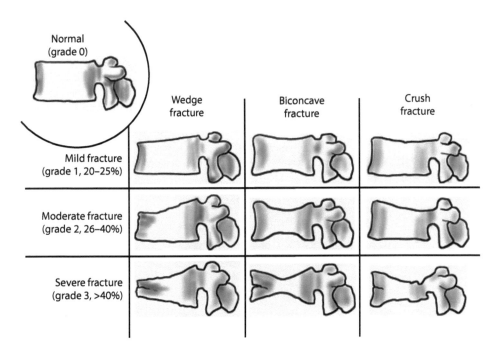

Figure 8.2. Genant classification for vertebral fractures
Reprinted by permission from Springer. Lasanianos, N.G., Triantafyllopoulos, G.K. and Pneumaticos, S.G. (2015) Osteoporotic Vertebral Fractures. In Lasanianos, N., Kanakaris, N. and Giannoudis, P. (eds) *Trauma and Orthopaedic Classifications.*

8.2.3 Blood tests

Blood tests for the investigation of osteoporosis should be performed at the initial assessment. They include the following:
- Calcium phosphate and vitamin D levels
- Renal function
- Thyroid function
- Parathyroid hormone levels
- Bone turnover markers, including type II collagen (CTX-II) and procollagen type 1 (P1NP)
- A myeloma screen may need to be considered in some patients.

Results showing abnormalities should be aimed at treating the underlying cause, thereby preventing further ongoing risk of osteoporosis.

8.2.4 FRAX tool

The FRAX (fracture risk algorithm) tool has been designed to help clinicians discuss with patients their individual risk of predicting the ten-year probability of a fracture. It is particularly useful for assessing patients who are treatment-naïve, and can be used to evaluate patients for a drug holiday from bone protective agents. The tool includes parameters incorporating specific risk factors in individual patients, including age, gender, weight, and risk factors with or without the addition of femoral neck BMD. The tool then provides the clinician and the patient with the percentage likelihood of a major fracture in the next 10 years. The FRAX tool has been independently evaluated to be effective and is approved by NICE in the UK and the Food and Drugs Administration in the USA (Kanis, 2002; www.sheffield.ac.uk/FRAX/tool.aspx).

8.3 Causes

Bone is made up of minerals, including calcium salts, with the whole structure being bound together by collagen fibres. Bone structure consists of a firm outer shell, called cortical or compact bone. The cortical bone is easily visible on plain X-rays. Deeper inside the bone there is a softer, spongy mesh of bone which has a honeycomb-like structure, called trabecular bone. Bone has a rich blood supply and is continually renewing itself. New bone is produced by cells called osteoblasts. Old bone tissue is broken down by cells called osteoclasts. There is a continual balance between anabolic and catabolic processes which build and break down bone, respectively.

During growth in childhood and adolescence, bone is formed rapidly and this allows bones to grow in length and become denser and stronger. Bone density reaches a peak by the mid- to late 20s. After age 40, bone starts to be broken down more rapidly than it is replaced, therefore bone density begins to fall. The rate of bone loss after age 40 determines whether someone will develop osteopenia/osteoporosis. The risk factors described in *Section 8.2* can all contribute to accelerated bone loss. Management of underlying risk factors will help prevent the progression of osteoporosis and the development of fractures (see *Figure 8.3*).

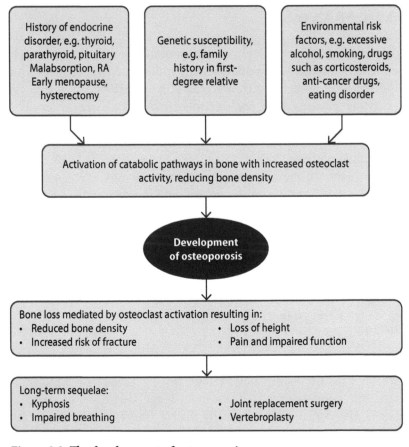

Figure 8.3. The development of osteoporosis

One of the earliest signs of osteoporosis can be the development of a fracture following a minor fall or accident, also known as a fragility or low impact fracture. The most common sites of fragility fractures include the hip, spine and wrist. Some patients may develop back pain if the vertebrae lose height and become weak, which results from the development of vertebral crush fractures. The regions most commonly affected include the mid- or lower back and such fractures can often happen without any fall or injury. If crush fractures occur in several regions, they can cause a curvature in the spine, with loss of height, also known as kyphosis. In some cases, crush fractures can cause difficulty in breathing and impairment of mobility.

8.4 Management

Management of osteoporosis is multidisciplinary and involves diet, exercise and pharmacological interventions, as discussed below. The management pathway is based on recommendations in the NICE guidelines, summarised in *Figure 8.4*.

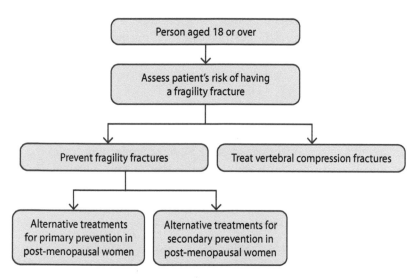

Figure 8.4. Assessing and managing fracture risk
Adapted from the NICE guidelines: https://cks.nice.org.uk/osteoporosis-prevention-of-fragility-fractures

8.4.1 Non-pharmacological interventions

Diet

It is important to establish from the patient their dietary intake of calcium and vitamin D. Calcium is naturally found in many products such as milk, yoghurt and cheese. Vitamin D is processed by the body in response to UVB in sunlight and is also present in certain foods, e.g. oily fish, red meat, liver and egg yolks. Active 1,25-dihydroxycholecalciferol, the active ingredient of vitamin D used by the body, requires hydroxylation in the liver and kidneys. People with certain dietary requirements, e.g. vegans, or those unable to tolerate dairy products, which are a rich source of calcium, may find it difficult to achieve the recommended daily intake. Others (e.g. those with eating disorders) may also be avoiding calcium and vitamin D. Numerous supplements are available for increasing dietary intake. Before starting treatment, levels of calcium and vitamin D should be checked in the serum. For vitamin D, serum ranges that help in guiding treatment are as follows: 25-hydroxyvitamin D levels, deficient (<25nmol/L), low to normal (25–50nmol/L) and sufficient (>50nmol/L) (see Royal Osteoporosis Society guidelines). For calcium, a corrected value is typically 2.2–2.6mmol/L. Further information on supplementation for low calcium and vitamin D levels is provided in *Table 8.5*.

Exercise

Weight-bearing exercise is essential for maintaining bone health. Exercises including walking, cycling and running are all invaluable in helping maintain bone density. Recommendations for exercise should be balanced with reducing the risk of falls, particularly in elderly people with osteopenia/osteoporosis who are at increased risk of falls. Many local services provide bone health classes and group exercise sessions for maintaining activity.

The Royal Osteoporosis Society has issued the 'Strong, Steady, Straight' statement which recommends physical activity and exercise for patients with osteoporosis based around improving bone strength, reducing falls and a focus on spine care whilst bending, moving and lifting.

8.4.2 Nutritional supplementation

Calcium and vitamin D

Depending on results from blood tests, it may be necessary to prescribe oral vitamin D and/or calcium supplementation. Examples of typical doses prescribed are shown in *Table 8.5*. In patients who only require vitamin D, this can be prescribed in varying doses depending on the level of deficiency. Blood tests can be checked in 2–3 months to check that patients are replete. It is often recommended to continue to take vitamin D supplements in those who are prone to deficiency, since levels tend to dip, particularly in winter months when sunlight is less and there is less natural ability of the body to hydroxylate vitamin D to its active form.

8.4.3 Disease-modifying therapies for osteoporosis

Bisphosphonates

Bisphosphonate drugs have been approved by NICE for treating osteoporosis. They inhibit osteoclast activity in osteoporosis, thereby preventing further deterioration of bone density. In some cases, with regular use over several years, bone density can also improve on bisphosphonates. A wide variety of formulations and treatments are available, which can be used depending on the clinical indication and individual patient needs. Different types of bisphosphonates are summarised in *Table 8.5*.

Key points for the use of bisphosphonates are as follows:
- Oral bisphosphonates, e.g. alendronic acid, ibandronic acid and risedronate sodium, are used as treatment for osteoporosis in adults if they have risk factors and the 10-year probability of osteoporotic fracture using the FRAX tool is high (see National Osteoporosis Guideline Group NOGG reference)
- IV bisphosphonates can be used to treat osteoporosis in adults when a person is at risk and has a 10-year probability of 10%, or the person has a probability risk of at least 1% but has difficulty taking oral bisphosphonates.

Important contraindications for the use of bisphosphonates include conception, pregnancy and breastfeeding, previous dental work

Table 8.5. Pharmacological management of osteoporosis

Drug	Formulation and dose	Mechanism of action	Usual level of therapy (NICE guidelines)	Screening	Monitoring
Vitamin D	PO Vitamin D3 400–1000 IU daily	Replenishes levels of vitamin D3, has anabolic effect on bone by increasing absorption of calcium	1st line	Check calcium, vitamin D, PTH levels	Calcium, vitamin D, PTH, FBC, U+Es, LFTs
Calcium and vitamin D	e.g. Calcichew D3 PO daily	Maintains vitamin D and calcium homeostasis and optimises anabolic bone metabolism	1st line	Check calcium, vitamin D, PTH levels	Calcium, vitamin D, PTH, FBC, U+Es, LFTs
Bisphosphonates	Alendronate 70mg PO weekly Zoledronate IV annually	Bisphosphonates bind to bone mineral, inhibiting osteoclast activity in bone through induction of osteoclast apoptosis	1st line	Check calcium, vitamin D, PTH levels Check dental history, renal function, check for history of osteonecrosis of the jaw/external auditory canal, atypical fractures, baseline DEXA scan	Calcium, vitamin D, PTH, FBC, U+Es, LFTs
Strontium ranelate	PO 2g once daily	It is a strontium salt of ranelic acid that increases deposition of new bone by osteoblasts and reduces resorption of bone by osteoclasts	2nd line	Check calcium, vitamin D, PTH levels at baseline, check for history of deep vein thrombosis, cerebrovascular disease, cardiovascular disease, uncontrolled hypertension	Calcium, vitamin D, PTH, FBC, U+Es, LFTs

Drug	Dose/route	Description	Line	Monitoring	Baseline tests
Denosumab	SC injection 60mg 6-monthly	High affinity humanised monoclonal antibody that binds to RANK ligand in bone. RANKL inhibition blocks osteoclast maturation, function and survival, thereby reducing bone resorption	2nd line	Check calcium, vitamin D, PTH levels at baseline, check for previous intolerance or adverse effects with bisphosphonates, cellulitis	Calcium, vitamin D, PTH, FBC, U+Es, LFTs
Raloxifene	PO 60mg daily	Raloxifene is a SERM which is a mixed agonist and antagonist of the oestrogen receptor in different tissues. It has oestrogenic activity in bone and increases bone mass. In the breast and uterine tissue it has anti-oestrogenic activity	2nd line	Check calcium, vitamin D, PTH levels at baseline, consider checking LH and FSH levels if appropriate to establish menopausal status	Calcium, vitamin D, PTH, FBC, U+Es, LFTs
Teriparatide	20 micrograms daily SC injection	Teriparatide is a synthetic form of parathyroid hormone containing 34 amino acids. It has anabolic effects on promoting bone formation in osteoporosis	2nd line	Check calcium, vitamin D, PTH levels at baseline, avoid if history of radiotherapy to the skeleton	Calcium, vitamin D, PTH, FBC, U+Es, LFTs
Calcitonin	100 units daily SC or IM	Inhibitor of osteoclast activity in bone	2nd line	Check calcium, vitamin D, PTH levels at baseline	Calcium, vitamin D, PTH, FBC, U+Es, LFTs

Abbreviations: FSH, follicle-stimulating hormone; LH, luteinising hormone; PTH, parathyroid hormone; RANK, receptor activator of nuclear factor kappa-B; SERM, selective oestrogen receptor modulator.

which may place the person at risk of avascular necrosis of the jaw, renal impairment and previous use of bisphosphonates. The drugs are usually prescribed for a period of 3–5 years, since increased benefit of bisphosphonates is not observed beyond this time period. The drug can be stopped early if there are adverse effects, e.g. jaw necrosis, renal impairment, GI side-effects, persistent flu-like symptoms.

Denosumab

Denosumab has been recommended by NICE. It is the first biologic which is being used to manage osteoporosis and is an inhibitor of RANKL (receptor activator of nuclear factor kappa-B ligand) in bone. It is usually used in post-menopausal women at increased risk of fractures who are unable to take bisphosphonates due to intolerance or contraindication and who have established risk factors for osteoporosis. Denosumab is recommended as a treatment option for the primary prevention of osteoporotic fragility fractures only in post-menopausal women at increased risk of fractures. It should not be stopped suddenly since sudden cessation can lead to increased fracture risk.

Raloxifene

The selective oestrogen receptor modulator (SERM) raloxifene is recommended in primary prevention of fragility fractures in post-menopausal women who have osteoporosis. In women aged ≥75 years, it can also be used without a DEXA scan if the scan is clinically inappropriate or unfeasible. The calcium and vitamin D levels should be corrected with supplementation if needed, before starting raloxifene.

Teriparatide

Teriparatide is a synthetic form of parathyroid hormone consisting of 34 amino acids. It has an anabolic effect, promoting bone formation in osteoporosis. It can be used in men and women. It is usually used when other agents have been inadequate at preventing fragility fractures and promoting bone formation. It can be used for up to two years.

Calcitonin

Calcitonin is a hormone which is naturally produced in the thyroid gland. It inhibits osteoclast activity in bone. It is administered intranasally and is usually used if other treatments, e.g. bisphosphonates, have not been effective in controlling osteoporosis and fragility fractures.

8.4.4 Vertebroplasty

Percutaneous vertebroplasty and percutaneous balloon kyphoplasty are not recommended by NICE for treating osteoporotic vertebral compression fractures in usual practice. However, vertebroplasty can be performed soon after vertebral compression fractures have developed, particularly for severe ongoing pain after a recent, unhealed vertebral fracture despite optimal pain management and in a patient whose pain has been confirmed at the level of the fracture by physical examination.

8.5 Cases

The following cases are based on real patients and are presented to help you consider how you would manage the scenarios.

Case history 8.1

A 54-year-old lady with RA is seen at her routine follow-up appointment in the Rheumatology department. Her arthritis is relatively well controlled and she has been on methotrexate 20mg weekly for the last 6 years. She had a DEXA scan to assess her bone density, as she had been experiencing menopausal symptoms for the last 6 months. Her DEXA scan results are shown below.

Bone density results				
Region	BMD (g/cm²)	T-score	Z-score	Classification
AP spine (L1–L4)	0.577	–4.3	–2.3	Osteoporosis
Femoral neck (left)	0.438	–3.7	–2.0	Osteoporosis
Total hip (left)	0.510	–3.5	–2.2	Osteoporosis
Femoral neck (right)	0.412	–3.9	–2.3	Osteoporosis
Total hip (right)	0.417	–4.3	–2.9	Osteoporosis

World Health Organization criteria for BMD impression classify patients as normal (T-score at or above –1.0), with osteopenia (T-score between –1.0 and –2.5) or osteoporosis (T-score at or below –2.5).

What treatment would you recommend for the patient?

- Strontium ranelate
- Alendronate
- Denosumab
- Teriparatide
- Calcitonin

Her DEXA scan shows osteoporosis. The patient is already taking calcium and vitamin D supplements. She is therefore likely to require bisphosphonate treatment. She is counselled for the treatment, including side-effects such as osteonecrosis of the jaw. After a dental check, she starts on alendronate 70mg orally weekly. She is advised about sitting upright for 30 minutes after taking the medication, to prevent reflux and abdominal discomfort.

Case history 8.2

An 84-year-old lady who lives in a nursing home is admitted to hospital after a fall from her chair in the nursing home. On admission to hospital, she is found to have a fractured neck of femur. She undergoes urgent surgery resulting in a right total hip replacement. Her X-ray of the hips and pelvis shows severe osteopenia. When she recovers from surgery, she reports that she had broken her wrist before the current admission, and her hospital records show she had a previous scaphoid fracture. She has dyspepsia and a previous duodenal ulcer, for which she has been on regular omeprazole. She is not well enough to undergo DEXA scanning. She is found to have low vitamin D levels in hospital, with normal calcium and parathyroid hormone levels. After 2 weeks of rehabilitation, she is deemed safe for discharge back to the nursing home.

What treatment should be organised in the long term?

- IV zoledronate once yearly
- SC denosumab 6-monthly
- Continue with vitamin D supplements only
- Start raloxifene
- Start calcitonin

Fragility fractures are common in post-menopausal women and this patient has already had two. Since she has dyspepsia and a previous duodenal ulcer, she would be suitable for IV zoledronate, which can be given annually.

Case history 8.3

A 70-year-old male had been treated with long-term corticosteroids for chronic obstructive pulmonary disease. He had been prescribed the bisphosphonate alendronate 70mg weekly for bone protection. He developed sudden thoracic back pain which also persisted at night. His GP arranged plain X-rays of the vertebral spine, which showed vertebral compression fractures at thoracic levels 7, 8 and 9. He also had blood tests which showed a normal renal and bone profile, normal parathyroid hormone levels, a normal myeloma screen and prostate-specific antigen. He had a DEXA scan which showed a T-score at the hip of −3.5 and −3.6 at the spine.

What would be the next best treatment option for him?

- Intravenous zoledronate
- Subcutaneous denosumab
- Subcutaneous teriparatide
- Continue oral alendronate
- Calcitonin

The best treatment option for a patient who has had treatment failure after 5 years of alendronate would be to switch to subcutaneous teriparatide. Teriparatide has a distinct mode of action compared with bisphosphonates, it is anabolic in action and is licensed for steroid-induced osteoporosis.

Case history 8.4

A 30-year-old woman is referred to the Rheumatologist by her GP. She had anorexia as a teenager and was diagnosed with hyperthyroidism in her twenties. She is currently taking carbimazole. She sustained a recent fall while riding her bicycle and was diagnosed as having a scaphoid fracture and a spinal fracture at T10. A DEXA scan confirmed osteoporosis at the spine and osteopenia at the hip. She reports that she follows a vegan diet and does not have any dairy in her diet. Blood tests show her vitamin D is <10nmol/L, calcium (corrected) is 2.36mmol/L, phosphate 0.9mmol/L, with normal thyroid function tests.

What treatment would you advise next?

- Vitamin D replacement
- Calcium supplementation
- Vitamin D replacement followed by calcium and vitamin D supplementation
- Vitamin D supplements

Since this lady is vitamin D deficient, she will first require vitamin D replacement e.g. with 20 000 IU orally per week for 12 weeks. Since she is a vegan, in the long term she is likely to require supplementation with calcium and vitamin D, e.g. Adcal D3 (chewable tablets), 400 units cholecalciferol and calcium 600mg per tablet, 2 tablets daily (800 units D3).

Case history 8.5

A 76-year-old woman with osteoporosis presents to her GP with thoracic back pain. She has previously been diagnosed with osteoporosis after she had a DEXA scan aged 60 years. She has taken calcium and vitamin D continuously for several years. She was started on alendronate but developed severe GI upset and stopped taking it. Spinal X-rays arranged by the GP show two wedge compression fractures at the level of T11 and T12.

What treatment would you advise next?

- Calcium supplementation
- Switch to risedronate
- Raloxifene
- Vitamin D supplementation
- Calcium and vitamin D

This patient would be suitable for raloxifene. She is post-menopausal and has confirmed fragility fractures on spinal X-rays. She has not been able to tolerate bisphosphonates and despite taking calcium and vitamin D supplements, she has still had fractures. It would therefore be reasonable for her to start an alternative bone modulator with a distinct mechanism of action.

8.6 References

Kanis, J.A. (2002) Diagnosis of osteoporosis and assessment of fracture risk. *Lancet*, **359:** 1929–36.

Kanis, J.A., Johnell, O., de Laet, C. *et al.* (2002) International variations in hip fracture probabilities: implications for risk assessment. *Journal of Bone & Mineral Research*, 17: 1237–1244.

Lasanianos, N.G., Triantafyllopoulos, G.K. and Pneumaticos, S.G. (2014) 'Osteoporotic Vertebral Fractures' in *Trauma and Orthopaedic Classifications*, pp. 251–254. SpringerLink.

National Osteoporosis Guideline Group (NOGG): www.sheffield.ac.uk/NOGG/mainrecommendations.html

World Health Organization (1994) *Assessment of fracture risk and its implication to screening for postmenopausal osteoporosis: Technical report series 843.* WHO.

NICE guidelines and useful websites

NICE guidelines for Osteoporosis management:

NICE 2014 (updated 2017), CG146; 2008 (updated 2011), TA160 and TA161; 2017, TA 464. www.nice.org.uk/guidance/conditions-and-diseases/diabetes-and-other-endocrinal--nutritional-and-metabolic-conditions/osteoporosis

NICE guidelines for prevention of fragility fractures: https://cks.nice.org.uk/osteoporosis-prevention-of-fragility-fractures

Royal Osteoporosis Society guidelines for vitamin D: www.guidelines.co.uk/musculoskeletal-and-joints-/ros-vitamin-d-and-bone-health-guideline/454558.article

Royal Osteoporosis Society physical activity and exercise for osteoporosis: https://theros.org.uk/media/0o5h1l53/ros-strong-steady-straight-quick-guide-february-2019.pdf

Sheffield FRAX tool: www.sheffield.ac.uk/FRAX/tool.aspx

CHAPTER 9

Chronic pain disorders

9.1 Introduction

It is estimated that chronic pain affects one-third to half of the UK population at any one time (Fayaz *et al.*, 2016). Among the most prevalent causes of chronic pain, musculoskeletal disorders feature highly. Fibromyalgia is one of the most frequent causes of chronic pain, estimated to affect 3–6% of the world population. It is most frequent in women, with 75–90% of cases being diagnosed in women. It can also affect men and children. Other disorders which have pain as a major symptom include different forms of arthritis, neuropathic pain (e.g. due to spinal disorders), regional pain syndromes, hypermobility disorders and reflex sympathetic dystrophy.

9.2 Diagnosis

Several diagnostic criteria have been developed for the diagnosis of chronic pain disorders. It is expected that symptom duration has been at least 3 months at a similar level of pain for a diagnosis to be made. Additional features required to make a diagnosis include pain localised to ≥4 out of 5 body regions (see *Figure 9.1*) and significant levels of pain on the fibromyalgia pain assessment score (Wolfe *et al.*, 2016). Additional features include sleep disturbance, fatigue throughout the day, multisite pain and hypersensitivity. More recent recommendations have proposed that a diagnosis of fibromyalgia is valid, regardless of other pre-existing diagnoses. Fibromyalgia can coexist in the presence of other chronic conditions, such as RA, back pain and SLE.

The following are features of fibromyalgia:
- Chronic widespread pain or multiple site pain for more than 3 months
- Cognitive problems
- Fatigue
- Sleep disturbance
- Other symptoms including headaches, abdominal pain, bloating, dizziness and paraesthesias
- Widespread soft tissue tenderness on clinical examination.

9.2.1 Blood tests

Blood tests are often performed to investigate for any other underlying cause of the symptoms, as follows:

ESR and CRP

It is useful to check inflammatory markers. They are often normal in fibromyalgia. Inflammatory markers are usually elevated in autoimmune inflammatory conditions such as RA or SLE.

Autoantibodies

It is common practice to check for autoantibodies, including ANA, RhF and anti-CCP.

Thyroid function tests

These are often performed to exclude physical causes of fatigue and systemic symptoms.

Full blood count

This is checked to ensure the subject does not have anaemia, which could be causing fatigue.

9.2.2 Imaging

Plain radiographs of affected regions are often performed and are likely to be normal in fibromyalgia. Other patients may have a CT chest if they have upper body pain, which is also often normal. For new diagnosis, it is often important to perform imaging to exclude any other serious underlying organic pathology. If there are other underlying conditions, e.g. RA, subjects may have radiographic changes consistent with those conditions, such as erosions and joint space narrowing.

Research in fibromyalgia using brain imaging studies suggests that people with chronic pain disorders have activation of pain networks in their brain with altered levels of neurotransmitters such as glutamate and dopamine. The activation of central brain pain networks in conditions such as fibromyalgia is also known as central sensitisation.

9.2.3 Pain measures

It is important to record consistent measures of pain in chronic pain disorders. There are several reasons for this. First, it provides a sequential record of how pain changes in individual subjects over time and how pain responses are altered in response to particular interventions. Secondly, it is important to record patient-reported pain outcome measures and compare them with physician assessments, so that an effective management plan can be developed with the patient. Pain can be divided into individual components, including inflammatory and neuropathic pain, with specific questionnaires that can be used to measure individual components of pain, discussed further below.

Inflammatory pain

Inflammatory pain is pain that traditionally arises in response to a local injury, e.g. joint pain, with release of local inflammatory mediators including molecules such as prostaglandins, leucotrienes, histamine and cytokines. Such mediators are released locally and cause an inflammatory response, leading to processes such as swelling, redness and pain. Inflammatory pain can be assessed by examination of affected regions and also by asking patients to complete questionnaires such as the Visual Analog Scale (0–100 rating scale) and Likert scales for pain. Many specific conditions have pain scores that have been validated for assessment of pain, e.g. McGill Pain Questionnalre, Numerical Rating Scale for Pain (0–10), Chronic Pain Grade Scale (CPGS), and Short Form-36 Bodily Pain Scale (Hawker *et al.*, 2011).

Neuropathic pain

Neuropathic pain is traditionally described as pain which arises from the central nervous system itself. It includes conditions such as spinal injuries that lead to spinal or back pain, and spinal cord injuries. Typical features of neuropathic pain include heightened pain sensitivity and allodynia. Allodynia refers to the phenomenon of heightened pain perception to a normal stimulus. Clinical examination can assess some features of neuropathic pain, e.g. allodynia and sensitisation. Questionnaires can also be used as part of the assessment; for example, the PAINDETECT questionnaire (Freynhagen *et al.*, 2006) includes a mannequin that allows patients to mark which area of the body is experiencing pain and also to describe more details about the nature of the pain, e.g. sharp, episodic, pins and needles. The PAINDETECT questionnaire provides a numerical score (0–35) which can be used to divide pain features into inflammatory and neuropathic components. Although initially developed to assess back pain, the questionnaire has now been used much more widely to assess different causes of neuropathic pain.

9.3 Causes

Fibromyalgia is a form of chronic pain disorder. For many years it was considered to be a psychological disorder. The cause of fibromyalgia is not fully understood. More recent brain imaging studies using functional MRI have shown that pain processing is altered in people with fibromyalgia. The brain imaging studies have shown that there are increased responses by certain brain regions to painful stimuli, so that people have heightened perception to pain, sometimes known as central sensitisation.

Risk factors for fibromyalgia which are non-modifiable include genetic factors, female sex and the presence of other painful conditions. Twin studies have suggested that the estimated heritability of chronic widespread pain is approximately 50%. People diagnosed with fibromyalgia are also more likely to have other painful conditions. A past medical history of depression, anxiety or previous abuse (e.g. physical) are also recognised risk factors for fibromyalgia. A summary of the causes of fibromyalgia is shown in *Figure 9.1.*

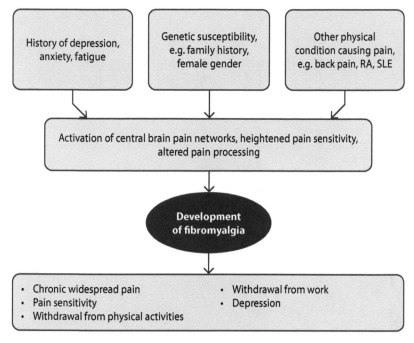

Figure 9.1. The development of fibromyalgia

9.4   Management

9.4.1 Non-pharmacological

Non-pharmacological treatments for fibromyalgia include graded exercises to build physical activity. Some services offer a rolling programme over several weeks as part of a pain management programme (PMP) that can identify patient needs, e.g. trying to improve sleep patterns and quality, pacing activities throughout the day and physical strengthening and activity.

Cognitive behavioural therapy (CBT) can be a significant part of a rehabilitation programme for fibromyalgia and other pain disorders. Some CBT programmes are delivered face-to-face, whereas others can be online, depending on patient preference.

Table 9.1. Pharmacological treatment of musculoskeletal pain disorders

Drug	Formulation and dose	Mechanism of action	Usual level of therapy (NICE guidelines)	Screening	Monitoring
Opioids	PO Typically e.g. codeine and paracetamol 15/500 up to 8 tablets daily	Inhibition of opioid-mediated pain pathways	1st line	No previous side-effects, respiratory problems, constipation	FBC, U+Es, LFTs
Capsaicin	Topical 0.025–0.05 micrograms	Modulates TRPV channels around skin and joint	1st line	Check for any skin rash	Monitor for allergic skin reactions
Tricyclic antidepressants (TCAs)	PO Typically amitriptyline 10mg nocte, dose can be increased	Inhibition of uptake of biogenic amines, e.g. noradrenaline	1st line	Any cardiac problems, e.g. arrhythmias, or previous intolerance to TCAs	Dry mouth, blurred vision, constipation, urinary retention
Serotonin–noradrenaline reuptake inhibitors (SNRIs)	PO Typically duloxetine 60mg daily	Inhibition of reuptake of serotonin and noradrenaline centrally	2nd line	Previous use of SNRIs or intolerance	Monitor for drowsiness, weight gain, unsteadiness, GI side-effects
Gabapentinoids	PO Typically gabapentin 300mg daily, can be increased or Pregabalin 150mg daily, can be increased	Modulation of GABAergic pathways in the CNS	2nd line	Previous use of gabapentinoids or intolerance	Monitor for drowsiness, unsteadiness, GI side-effects

9.4.2 Pharmacological

A variety of analgesic medications targeting specific pathways can be used to treat pain disorders. The main classes of drugs used are summarised in *Table 9.1*.

9.5 Other pain disorders

Several other disorders which cause chronic pain commonly present to musculoskeletal services. The most prevalent disorders are described below.

9.5.1 Complex regional pain syndrome

Complex regional pain syndrome (CRPS) is a condition which causes severe chronic pain which can be very debilitating. Many cases are triggered by an injury, which then leads to heightened pain sensitivity and pain in the long term. It can occur at any age from childhood to adulthood, but most commonly affects women between the ages of 60 and 70. The prevalence ranges between 6 and 26 per 100 000 patient years, with an increased likelihood of it affecting the upper limbs to the lower limbs in a ratio of 3:2. Diagnosis is based on history, e.g. trauma such as surgery or an accident resulting in crush injuries or fractures and clinical examination, which may reveal colour changes in the skin, hypersensitivity, changes in nail and hair growth patterns, and impaired movement. Management includes providing clear information to the patient about self-management, physical rehabilitation including physiotherapy, pain relief (see *Figure 10.3*) and psychological support, which may include CBT. Physiotherapy aims to restore as much normal function as possible and to improve quality of life. Graded image therapy is often used with the aim to 'retrain' the way the brain interacts with the limbs.

9.5.2 Hypermobility

Hypermobility syndrome is a common set of disorders which have an estimated prevalence of 1 in 5000 worldwide. The female to male ratio is estimated at 3:1. The main symptoms are pain or stiffness in the joints or muscles, recurrent injuries such as joint dislocations or sprains, poor balance and coordination, thin, stretchy skin and some GI problems such as diarrhoea or constipation. The genetic basis of hypermobility includes mutations in type II collagen fibril formation, and a wide variety of mutations are recognised. Some people can experience chronic widespread pain as a result of this condition. Severe cases are also associated with anxiety and depression.

An important aspect of management includes providing clear information about the condition to the patient, goal setting, pacing, physiotherapy, pain relief (see *Table 9.1*) and psychological support, which may include CBT.

9.6 Cases

The following cases are based on real patients and are presented to help you consider how you would manage the scenarios.

Case history 9.1

A 55-year-old lady is referred to the Rheumatology clinic with widespread pain symptoms. She has experienced pain and stiffness in her shoulders for several years. She was initially told she had rotator cuff disease and had physiotherapy, which worked for a few months; however, her symptoms have now recurred. She now has intermittent chest pains and back pain. She has difficulty sleeping at night and wakes up several times a night with pain. The GP has also diagnosed her with depression and recently started her on citalopram, which has helped to a certain extent. She is finding it difficult to cope. She has already tried co-codamol 15/500 up to 6 tablets per day but still has ongoing pain.

She is examined by the Rheumatologist who finds multiple tender points on physical examination including the anterior chest, shoulders, thoracic and spinal regions posteriorly. She also has allodynia.

What investigations would be helpful?

- ESR
- Thyroid function tests
- X-ray spine and shoulders
- CT brain
- CRP

At first assessment, it is useful to exclude any other underlying disorder such as an inflammatory condition, OA or thyroid disease. The patient does not have any suggestion of organic brain symptoms, so a CT brain would not be indicated.

All her investigations are normal and a diagnosis of fibromyalgia is made. She is referred to the PMP, which includes CBT, advice on taking analgesic medication and pacing. After 6 months she is reviewed in clinic. She is much improved and is sleeping better. She remains under review with the GP.

Case history 9.2

An 18-year-old female is seen in her GP surgery. She has developed chronic pain in her legs and is unable to walk without using crutches. She has also been taking paracetamol regularly due to pain in her legs. She feels very depressed and helpless as she was due to start university soon. She used to be very active as a child and was involved in gymnastics at regional competitions. Her GP arranges blood tests, including a FBC, autoantibody screen, inflammatory markers including ESR/CRP, thyroid, renal and liver function tests, all of which are normal. X-rays of the lower limbs are also normal. The GP refers the patient urgently to a Rheumatologist. On further questioning, the patient reports that her mother suffers from Ehlers–Danlos syndrome. She also recalls that she had a shoulder dislocation aged 15. The Rheumatologist examines the patient. On examination, the patient has several features of hypermobility syndrome, particularly in her lower limbs, with a Beighton score of 5/9.

What treatment should the patient have next?

- Increase analgesia with prescription of opiates
- Start antidepressant medication
- Refer patient for CBT
- Refer patient for physiotherapy
- Discharge the patient with an exercise sheet

Although there is no cure for joint hypermobility syndrome, due to often pre-existing abnormalities e.g. in collagen II fibres in connective tissues, several interventions have been shown to be of benefit in hypermobility syndrome. These include physiotherapy, for specialist advice on improving muscle strength and fitness so that the joints are protected. The aims of physiotherapy are to reduce pain and the risk of dislocations, and to improve muscle strength, posture and balance.

9.7 References

Fayaz, A., Croft, P., Langford, R.M. *et al.* (2016) Prevalence of chronic pain in the UK: a systematic review and meta-analysis of population studies. *BMJ Open*, **6:** e010364.

Freynhagen, R., Baron, R., Gockel, U. and Tölle, T.R. (2006) painDETECT: a new screening questionnaire to identify neuropathic components in patients with back pain. *Curr Med Res Opin.*, **22(10):** 1911–20.

Hawker, G.A., Mian, S., Kendzerska, T. and French, M. (2011) Measures of adult pain: Visual Analog Scale for Pain (VAS Pain), Numeric Rating Scale for Pain (NRS Pain), McGill Pain Questionnaire (MPQ), Short-Form McGill Pain Questionnaire (SF-MPQ), Chronic Pain Grade Scale (CPGS), Short Form-36 Bodily Pain Scale (SF-36 BPS), and Measure of Intermittent and Constant Osteoarthritis Pain (ICOAP). *Arthritis Care Res.*, **63 Suppl 1:** S240–52.

Macfarlane, G.J., Kronisch, C., Dean, L.E. *et al.* (2017) EULAR revised recommendations for the management of fibromyalgia. *Ann Rheumatic Dis.*, **76:** 318–328.

Wolfe, F., Clauw, D.J., Fitzcharles, M-A. *et al.* (2016) 2016 Revisions to the 2010/2011 fibromyalgia diagnostic criteria. *Semin Arthritis Rheum.*, **46(3):** 319–329.

Useful websites for patient support

www.awaywithpain.co.uk/

https://painuk.org/

Exercises to manage pain:
www.versusarthritis.org/about-arthritis/managing-symptoms/exercise/exercises-to-manage-pain/

www.versusarthritis.org/about-arthritis/conditions/complex-regional-pain-syndrome-crps/

www.hypermobility.org/what-are-hypermobility-syndromes

10

Soft tissue disorders

10.1 Introduction

Soft tissue disorders encompass a variety of conditions, including tendinopathy, tendinitis, bursitis and in some cases, irreversible damage to soft tissues such as shoulder rotator cuff tears and labral tears.

In this chapter we will discuss rotator cuff pathology as an exemplar for managing soft tissue conditions. Rotator cuff pathology encompasses numerous pathologies including tendinopathy, tendinitis, bursitis and rotator cuff tears. The term commonly used for all these conditions is 'rotator cuff-related shoulder pain'. Shoulder conditions have a UK prevalence of 14%. Rotator cuff pathology can account for up to 70% of all shoulder conditions. Those affected are commonly between the ages of 35 and 75 years; both men and women are affected. Pain is a predominant feature, especially with overhead activities, reaching behind the back, and sleeping on the affected side. Patients may present with weakness.

10.2 Diagnosis

Ensuring the correct diagnosis is paramount and will ensure the patient is managed appropriately. The algorithm in *Figure 10.1*, developed by Rees and Carr (Kulkarni *et al.*, 2015), highlights other shoulder pathologies and provides guidelines on treatment and referral. Structures around the shoulder which can give rise

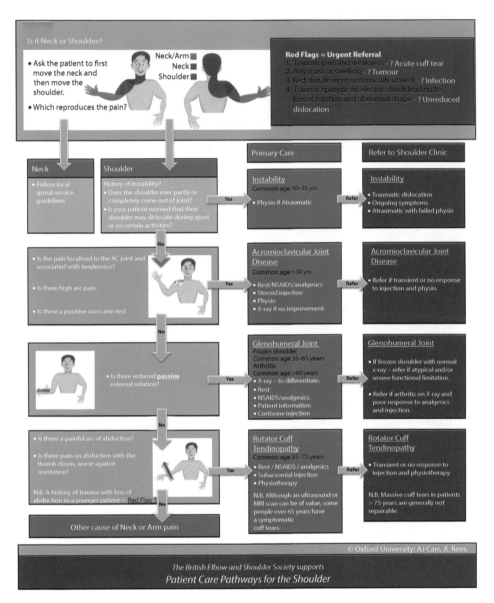

Figure 10.1. Diagnosis of shoulder problems in primary care. Guidelines on treatment and referral

Reproduced from Kulkarni, R., Gibson, J., Brownson, P. *et al.* (2015) BESS/BOA Patient Care Pathways: subacromial shoulder pain. *Shoulder & Elbow*, **7(2)**: 135–143; SAGE, with permission.

to shoulder pain include the cervical spine, thoracic outlet and biceps tendon, which can be part of underlying conditions such as rheumatoid arthritis and osteoarthritis.

Any 'red flags' highlighted during a primary care assessment need urgent secondary care referral. For shoulder conditions, these include the following:

- Suspected joint infection
- Unreduced dislocation
- Suspected tumour or malignancy – urgent referral following the local 2-week cancer referral pathway
- Acute cuff tear as a result of trauma
- Shoulder pain with symptoms suggestive of a systemic inflammatory joint disease should be referred into Rheumatology via local referral pathways.

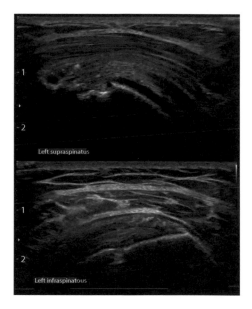

Figure 10.2. Ultrasound shoulder showing rotator cuff disease
Extensive irregular echogenicity involving the entire infraspinatus and posterior fibres of supraspinatus. The absence of associated acoustic shadowing is in keeping with type 2 tendon calcification. There is cortical irregularity and heterogeneous hypoechogenicity within the supraspinatus tendon.

10.2.1 Imaging

In the absence of any red flags or history of trauma, imaging is not indicated in primary care unless conservative management has been unsuccessful (www.bess.org.uk). There is growing evidence showing a lack of correlation between symptoms and rotator cuff integrity. Some studies found that up to 40% of the general population had asymptomatic rotator cuff tears. Any positive findings on imaging should be interpreted within the clinical context and a management plan based on patient needs and abilities. The most common imaging modalities include ultrasound and MRI, which can aid in defining the extent of involvement, e.g. tendinitis and the presence of tears (see *Figure 10.2*).

10.3 Causes

The aetiology of rotator cuff tendinopathy is multifactorial but proposed mechanisms in the literature include intrinsic, extrinsic or combined factors (*Figure 10.3*). Currently it has been recognised that the level of physical damage (e.g. tendinopathy, the presence of tears, bursitis, joint effusion) does not always directly correlate with the level of clinical symptoms, including altered function and pain. The level of pain varies greatly between individuals and the reasons for this are unclear. Several studies suggest that central sensitisation or cortical changes could be contributing, with pain not always being caused by local pathology.

10.4 Management

10.4.1 Non-pharmacological management

Physiotherapy

General principles of physiotherapy include the following:
• An individualised, holistic approach
• A patient-centred management programme

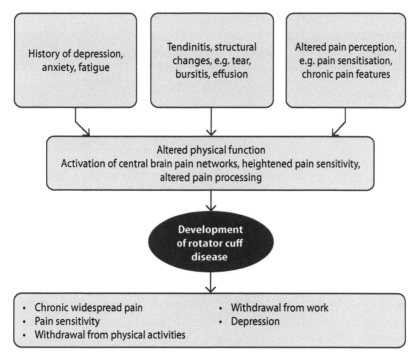

Figure 10.3. Development of rotator cuff disease

- Addressing functional impairment
- Tailoring management within the remit of the patient's lifestyle factors
- Identifying coping strategies within the patient's expectations and ability
- Recommending exercises that can be achieved while taking into consideration the patient's level of pain.

The consensus is that initial management should be conservative, as there is limited evidence that surgery is more effective than physiotherapy. A systematic review and meta-analysis (Saltychev et al., 2015) looked at conservative treatment versus surgery for shoulder impingement and found no significant difference. Physiotherapy is cost-effective and has reduced complications compared to surgery (Ketola, Lehtinen and Arnala, 2017). *Table 10.1* summarises the types of soft tissue disorders covered in this chapter and the appropriate physiotherapy exercises recommended.

Table 10.1. Physiotherapy for soft tissue disorders

Type of soft tissue disorder	Recommended exercises
Medial and lateral epicondylitis	www.youtube.com/watch?v=Lf695_IJO8g
Rotator cuff disease	https://bess.ac.uk/patient-care-pathways-and-guidelines/
	www.youtube.com/channel/UC09T_cXrnSFu-irWGcfEifg
Achilles, hamstring, patellar tendinitis	www.youtube.com/watch?v=GKkSp-Tlofl
	www.youtube.com/watch?v=EZUSKrZYBfc

The overall aim of physiotherapy treatment is to improve pain and function, with shared decision-making with the patient throughout. It is individual to each patient depending on their clinical assessment.

Patient education is essential to successful outcomes. It is important to provide reassurance to the patient that there is no serious injury or disease. Seek to address any fears and anxieties the patient may have. Work on patient-centred goals, taking into account the patient's expectations and their understanding of their condition. Try to encourage normal activities and self-management strategies. Explore other factors such as poor sleep, anxiety, depression and poor self-efficacy, which can also determine outcome. Educate patients on lifestyle factors such as smoking, stress and nutrition, which can influence outcomes.

It has been suggested that stages of rotator cuff tendinopathy can be subcategorised. These include irritable rotator cuff tendinopathy, non-irritable rotator cuff tendinopathy and degenerative rotator cuff tendinopathy. Each subgroup receives individualised treatment programmes, based around their clinical presentation.

Patients with irritable rotator cuff tendinopathy can present with constant pain, often at night and following minimal activity. Pain reduction is paramount at this stage. Incorporate relative rest and modify activities that exacerbate symptoms. An exercise diary may be helpful at this stage to identify any triggers to flare-ups. Injection therapy using intra-articular corticosteroids may be indicated in these patients. Physiotherapists can perform these injections. Although evidence is equivocal, subacromial bursa injections may be associated with more effective clinical outcomes.

Once irritability has settled, or in the non-irritable patient, scapular and rotator cuff exercises can be introduced in a graded programme. Rehabilitation should be specific and consideration should be given to the trunk and lower limb, as it plays an important part in patients' function and sport; evidence suggests exercise programmes should be carried out over a period of 6–12 weeks. General musculoskeletal fitness should also be included. Heron *et al.* (2017) found open chain, closed chain and range of motion exercises were effective in reducing pain and disability in the short term in patients with rotator cuff tendinopathy. Shire *et al.* (2017) conducted a systematic literature review and meta-analysis and found insufficient evidence to support or refute the effectiveness of specific resistive exercise strategies in the rehabilitation of subacromial pain. They concluded that more high quality research was needed, thus a general approach to exercise may be just as effective.

Ainsworth *et al.* (2009) developed a specific pathway for the management of massive non-operable rotator cuff repairs, which involves a progression of exercises from lying to sitting to standing. This is available online at www.bobbyainsworth.com.

10.4.2 Pharmacological management

If physiotherapy has not been effective, or there are ongoing pain symptoms, patients can be offered a corticosteroid injection. These can be done by experienced practitioners (e.g. trained GPs, physiotherapists) who are trained in injecting. There are specific regions of the shoulder associated with tendinitis which may benefit from injection, such as glenohumeral injections, and subacromial bursal injections. Injections can also be performed under ultrasound guidance, which is often instilled in combination with anaesthetic.

For longer-term pain management, topical anti-inflammatory NSAID gels can be used. Alternatives to this include capsaicin cream. In patients requiring stronger analgesia, oral NSAIDs and/or opioids can also be used. Patients should always be warned about side-effects, including peptic ulcer and GI upset with NSAIDs, constipation and drowsiness with opioids. If a patient requires long-term NSAIDs, a PPI should be prescribed to prevent development of peptic ulcer disease in the long term.

10.5 Other soft tissue disorders

Other regions which can be affected by tendinopathy and bursitis include the elbow. Commonly affected tendons in the elbow include the extensor and flexor tendons of the forearms. Patellar tendinopathy, or 'jumper's knee', is also common, particularly in people who do sports that involve jumping, such as basketball, netball or volleyball. Achilles tendinopathy also occurs frequently, and subjects should always be screened for any other evidence of inflammatory changes, since tendinopathy can be a feature of inflammatory conditions such as ankylosing spondylitis and psoriatic arthritis. Patients may also be suffering from Achilles tendinopathy related to mechanical overloading.

Diagnosis is often confirmed by clinical examination and imaging. Management follows the principles outlined in *Section 10.4*.

10.6 Cases

The following cases are based on real patients and are presented to help you consider how you would manage the scenarios.

Case history 10.1

A 24-year-old male rugby player who plays club level rugby presented to his GP with a 3-week history of shoulder pain after weightlifting in the gym. He felt a sudden onset of pain later that day which was worse the next morning. His symptoms are aggravated by shoulder abduction, hand behind back, and external rotation. No pins and needles, numbness, swelling, clunking, clicking and no previous injury were reported, nor any night pain.

What treatment would you recommend?

Physiotherapy is the first-line treatment for this patient. This would consist of advice and recommendation of modifying aggravating activities. It is important to promote relative rest in the early stages. Educate the patient regarding their condition (see the British Elbow & Shoulder Society (BESS) website, www.bess.ac.uk).

Modify aggravating activities and promote relative rest for rotator cuff disease. Educate the patient regarding his condition; continue to encourage cardiovascular training and kinetic chain work. Progress to functional loading and sport-specific rehabilitation, and look at weightlifting technique.

Case history 10.2

A 54-year-old secretary is seen by her GP. She has noticed pain in her right elbow which is worse when she is typing and cooking. She finds it difficult to carry her shopping bags without feeling pain. More recently she has been dropping objects. She has been taking ibuprofen 400mg regularly but is still experiencing pain. On examination she is found to have unilateral lateral tendinopathy, or 'tennis elbow'.

What is the next best treatment option?

- Physiotherapy
- PRP (platelet-rich plasma) injection
- Dry needling under US guidance
- Shock wave therapy

Physiotherapy is the first treatment of choice. In the initial stages 'relative rest' is advised through modification of provocative daily activities. The patient should be given ergonomic advice and eccentric tendon loading. Should physiotherapy not achieve optimal outcome, then shock wave therapy would be indicated. The next level of treatment would be dry needling followed by PRP injections. Although all options given are potential treatments that can be used for tennis elbow, most treatment plans usually start with physiotherapy. Physiotherapy provides exercises to help strengthen the flexor and extensor tendon insertions in the forearm and to prevent long-term chronic symptoms. Steroid injections are sometimes used in very resistant cases. If the condition becomes chronic and a US scan shows evidence of neovascularisation with chronic pain, dry needling can be performed under US guidance to alleviate symptoms.

Case history 10.3

A 30-year-old male has been training with his hockey team for a tournament. He develops severe pain and swelling in the knee. He is unable to run or jump for any sustained period and has stopped training. He is seen by the GP who examines his knee to find tenderness below the inferior margin of the patella but normal range of movement. He diagnoses the patient with patellar tendinopathy.

What treatment should be recommended?

- Intra-articular corticosteroid injection
- Dry needling procedure
- Shock wave therapy
- Physiotherapy
- Non-weight-bearing rest

The patient is referred for physiotherapy. He is given activity modification advice, a graded loading exercise programme and gradual sport-specific rehabilitation to perform over 6–8 weeks, in order for him to return to playing hockey. He is encouraged with cross-training exercises such as circuits, cycling and swimming. He gradually recovers and is able to play for his team again. Intra-articular corticosteroid injection and non-weight-bearing rest are not recommended for patellar tendinopathy.

10.7 References

Ainsworth, R., Lewis, J. and Conboy, V. (2009) A prospective randomized placebo controlled clinical trial of a rehabilitation programme for patients with a diagnosis of massive rotator cuff tears of the shoulder. *Shoulder and Elbow*, **1(1)**: 55–60.

Coronado, R.A., Seitz, A.L., Pelote, E. *et al.* (2018) Are psychosocial factors associated with patient-reported outcome measures in patients with rotator cuff tears? A systematic review. *Clin Orthop Relat Res.*, **476(4)**: 810–829.

Heron, S.R., Woby, S.R. and Thompson, D.P. (2017) Comparison of three types of exercise in the treatment of rotator cuff tendinopathy/shoulder impingement syndrome: a randomized controlled trial. *Physiotherapy*, **103(2)**: 167–173.

Ketola, S., Lehtinen, J.T. and Arnala, I. (2017) Arthroscopic decompression not recommended in the treatment of rotator cuff tendinopathy: a final review of a randomised controlled trial at a minimum follow-up of ten years. *Bone Joint J.*, **99-B(6)**: 799–805.

Kulkarni, R., Gibson, J., Brownson, P. *et al.* (2015) BESS/BOA Patient Care Pathways: subacromial shoulder pain. *Shoulder & Elbow*, **7(2)**: 135–143.

Lewis, J., McCreesh, K., Roy, J-S. and Ginn, K. (2015) Rotator cuff tendinopathy: navigating the diagnosis–management conundrum. *J Orthop Sports Phys Ther.*, **45(11)**: 923–937.

Saltychev, M., Äärimaa, V., Virolainen, P. and Laimi, K. (2015) Conservative treatment or surgery for shoulder impingement: systematic review and meta-analysis. *Disabil Rehabil.*, **37(1)**: 1–8.

Shire, A.R., Stæhr, T.A., Overby, J.B. *et al.* (2017) Specific or general exercise strategy for subacromial impingement syndrome – does it matter? A systematic literature review and meta-analysis. *BMC Musculoskelet Disord.*, **18(1)**: 158.

Useful websites

Shoulder assessment

Shoulder examination: www.youtube.com/watch?v=Po1WVWALKz0

NHS physiotherapy for shoulder pain: www.youtube.com/watch?v=XXwXJ1IAzxc

British Elbow and Shoulder Society website includes videos for patient shoulder exercises: https://bess.ac.uk/

Ask Dr Jo: '10 best rotator cuff exercises for strengthening': www.youtube.com/watch?v=6u8QpNmQy_g

Tennis and golfer's elbow

Lateral epicondylalgia exercises: www.youtube.com/watch?v=Lf695_IJO8g

Knee and back

'Tendinitis, tendinosis, tendiopathy? Exercise is the best medicine for tendon pain': www.youtube.com/watch?v=GKkSp-TlofI

Ask Dr Jo: 'Patellar tendonitis exercises & stretches for pain relief': www.youtube.com/watch?v=EZUSKrZYBfc

ESCAPE-pain: https://escape-pain.org

Exercise-focused apps and websites

Evidence-based digital app used in the NHS that is referred by GP or clinician prescribing physiotherapy exercises and providing self-management options for patients. Mainly for cervical spine and shoulder pain: www.getubetter.com

EXI provides general exercise suggested by healthcare professionals, where progress can be monitored: https://exi.life

NHS Live Well website: www.nhs.uk/live-well

Chartered Society of Physiotherapy website and leaflets; 'Love Activity, hate exercise' campaign: www.csp.org.uk/public-patient/keeping-active-and-healthy/love-activity-hate-exercise-campaign

Versus Arthritis Exercises for managing pain: www.versusarthritis.org/about-arthritis/managing-symptoms/exercise/exercises-to-manage-pain/

Couch to 5K, a recommended running plan for beginners: www.nhs.uk/live-well/exercise/couch-to-5k-week-by-week/

CHAPTER 11

Paediatric rheumatology

11.1 Introduction

Paediatric rheumatology covers a range of conditions which affect children and young people up to the age of 18 years. One of the commonest disorders presenting to paediatrics is juvenile idiopathic arthritis (JIA), which will be discussed in detail in this chapter. JIA has a prevalence of 1 in 1000 children, with an onset before the age of 16 and a symptom duration of at least 6 weeks. Girls are affected twice as commonly as boys.

11.2 Diagnosis

JIA can present with a variety of symptoms, including the following:
- Joint pain or stiffness, often most prominent in the early morning
- Painful, red, hot or swollen joints
- A child or young adult feeling very tired or run-down
- Blurred vision or dry, gritty eyes, due to uveitis
- Skin rash
- Loss of appetite
- High fever

11.2.1 Forms of JIA

JIA is classified into different forms, including the following:
- Oligoarthritis: affects ≤4 joints, typically large joints (knees, ankles, elbows). This is the most common subtype of JIA.

- Polyarthritis: affects ≥5 joints, often on both sides of the body (e.g. both knees, both wrists). May affect large and small joints. Affects approximately 25% of children with JIA.
- Systemic arthritis: affects the whole body (joints, skin and internal organs). Symptoms can include a high spiking fever which can last for >1 week and sometimes an associated rash. The systemic form affects approximately 10% of children with JIA.
- Psoriatic arthritis: joint symptoms include a rash in typical areas affected by psoriasis, including a scaly rash behind the ears, eyelids, elbows, umbilicus, scalp. The arthritis can affect ≥1 joints, including the wrists, knees, ankles, fingers or toes.
- Enthesitis-related JIA, due to spondyloarthritis: most prominently occurs where the muscles, ligaments or tendons attach to the bone, called the entheses. This form can affect the hips, knees and feet. More rarely it can also affect the fingers, pelvis, elbows, chest, digestive tract (e.g. Crohn's disease or ulcerative colitis) and lower back. Lower back involvement is classified as ankylosing spondylitis and is often associated with sacroiliitis, which is more common in boys, typically between the ages of 8 and 15.
- Temporomandibular joint arthritis: can occur in isolation in JIA and can impair growth of the jaw, eating and nutritional intake.
- Undifferentiated JIA: in this form the symptoms do not typically fit into any group, but inflammation is found in one or more joints.

11.2.2 Investigations

These are performed to investigate for the presence of inflammation and to exclude other disorders, e.g. anaemia, infection or malignancy.
- ESR: often elevated at presentation and during flares
- CRP: often elevated at presentation and during flares
- ANA: may be positive
- RhF: can be positive in JIA
- Anti-CCP antibodies: can be positive in JIA
- HLA-B27: this is associated with enthesitis-related forms, including ankylosing spondylitis
- Full blood count: to check for anaemia, white cell counts
- Imaging: may include plain radiographs of the affected joint, ultrasound or MRI scans – e.g. of the spine – to investigate specific signs and symptoms.

11.3 Causes

JIA is an autoimmune condition caused by dysregulation of the immune system. There is often evidence of autoimmunity detected by the presence of autoantibodies, e.g. ANA, RhF, anti-CCP antibodies. There is an increased recruitment of inflammatory cells into the joints, which causes inflammation in the synovium, or lining of the joint. Ongoing inflammation in the synovium leads to a joint becoming hot, painful, swollen and tender.

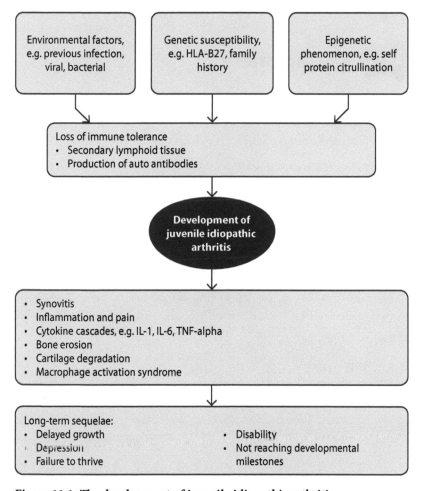

Figure 11.1. The development of juvenile idiopathic arthritis

Although the actual cause of JIA is not fully understood, it is known that infections can trigger the development of the condition, although in most cases the actual pathogen is not identified. Certain genetic risk factors, e.g. HLA-B27, are also known to be associated with some forms of JIA. The causes and consequences of JIA are summarised in *Figure 11.1*. In severe cases of systemic JIA, a complication called macrophage activation syndrome (MAS) can occur, where patients may have a very high ferritin level, with at least two of the following: low platelets, high triglycerides, high AST and low fibrinogen levels. MAS can require treatment with high dose corticosteroids, biologic agents targeted to interleukin-1, such as anakinra, and also support on intensive care (Ravelli *et al.*, 2016).

11.4 Management

There is no cure for JIA but remission, which helps to achieve little or no disease activity or symptoms, is possible. Early aggressive treatment is key to getting the disease under control as quickly as possible.

The goals of JIA treatment are to:
- slow down or stop inflammation
- relieve symptoms, control pain and improve quality of life
- prevent joint and organ damage
- preserve joint function and mobility
- reduce long-term health effects
- achieve remission (little or no disease activity or symptoms).

Treatment for JIA varies depending on disease type and severity. A well-rounded plan includes medication, complementary therapies and healthy lifestyle habits.

11.4.1 Exercise

Regular physical exercise can ease joint stiffness and pain, including low impact activities such as walking, swimming, cycling and yoga.

11.4.2 Physical therapies

Physical and occupational therapy can improve a child's quality of life. Children can learn ways to stay active and how to perform daily activities without pain. Physical and occupational therapists can teach and guide them through strengthening and flexibility exercises, with examples provided as follows:

- www.youtube.com/watch?v=iswHK1M_iik
- www.versusarthritis.org/media/1415/my-child-has-arthritis-booklet.pdf

In some cases, manipulation may be performed and assistive devices such as braces and splints provided.

11.4.3 Non-steroidal anti-inflammatory drugs

NSAIDs can be used to improve pain and relieve symptoms. However, they cannot reduce joint damage or change the course of JIA. Recommended doses in children are lower; for example, ibuprofen, which is one of the most commonly used NSAIDs in children, is typically used at a maximum dose of 30mg/kg per day. For specific drug doses on different NSAIDs in children, clinicians can refer to the British National Formulary (BNF) (www.bnf.org).

11.4.4 Disease-modifying antirheumatic drugs

DMARDs are often used to treat people with sustained symptoms. The most commonly used drug for JIA is methotrexate. Many patients' symptoms are controlled with methotrexate. However, if there is ongoing disease activity, biologics can be used to control the disease, including etanercept, adalimumab and tocilizumab. Drugs used are summarised in *Table 11.1*.

Table 11.1. Disease-modifying therapies used in the management of JIA (rows with light background are synthetic DMARDs; those with darker background are biologic DMARDs)

Drug	Formulation and dose	Mechanism of action	Usual level of therapy (NICE guidelines)	Screening	Monitoring
Methotrexate	PO/SC Typically 15–25mg weekly	Inhibition of purine synthesis	1st line	Hepatitis B & C, HIV	FBC, U+Es, LFTs
Sulfasalazine	PO Typically 1–3g daily in divided doses	Inhibitor of expression of TNF and other cytokines	1st line	Hepatitis B & C, HIV	FBC, U+Es, LFTs
Hydroxchloroquine	PO Up to 400mg daily in divided doses	Inhibitor of expression of TNF and other cytokines	1st line	Hepatitis B & C, HIV	FBC, U+Es, LFTs
Corticosteroids, e.g. prednisolone	PO/IM	Works through multiple pathways including increased transcription of anti-inflammatory genes	1st line	Monitor for diabetes, hypertension	FBC, U+Es, LFTs
Adalimumab (Humira)	40mg SC every 2 weeks	Humanised anti-TNF monoclonal antibody	2nd line	Hepatitis B & C, HIV	FBC, U+Es, LFTs
Etanercept (Enbrel, Benepali biosimilar)	50mg SC weekly or 25mg twice-weekly	TNF fusion protein	2nd line	Hepatitis B & C, HIV, TB	FBC, U+Es, LFTs
Tocilizumab (Actemra)	IV/SC every 4 weeks	Monoclonal antibody to IL-6 receptor	2nd line	Hepatitis B & C, HIV, TB	FBC, U+Es, LFTs, lipids
Abatacept (Orencia)	IV/SC (weekly if SC)	Fusion protein of IgG1 and CTLA-4	2nd line	Hepatitis B & C, HIV, TB	FBC, U+Es, LFTs

11.4.5 Surgery

DMARD therapies including methotrexate and biologics have significantly reduced the rates of surgery in children and young people with JIA.

In cases where DMARD therapies have been unable to fully control inflammation, joint damage and function, surgery may be indicated, e.g. hip or knee replacements, which are some of the most common joint surgeries in JIA.

11.5 Cases

The following cases are based on real patients and are presented to help you consider how you would manage the scenarios.

Case history 11.1

A 7-year-old girl presents with a limp for the last few weeks. Her mum reports that she has had red eyes for the last 4 weeks. She is seen in A&E. On examination there is swelling in the right knee with synovitis and an effusion. She has reduced range of movement with a positive patellar tap. Blood tests show she has an ESR of 45, CRP of 23 and she is ANA-positive. The girl is given oral ibuprofen regularly for 2 weeks and referred to the Paediatric Rheumatology clinic.

When she is seen in the clinic 4 weeks later her knee swelling has resolved. She has had one further episode of red eye and was given steroid eye drops by the GP, who diagnosed uveitis. The Consultant in the Paediatric Rheumatology clinic confirms the diagnosis with the girl and her family.

What is the most likely diagnosis?

- Oligoarticular JIA
- Systemic JIA
- Conjunctivitis
- Parvovirus infection
- Reactive arthritis

The girl has had symptoms for 8 weeks including uveitis with swelling and inflammation of her knee.

She also has signs of an inflammatory response with a raised ESR and CRP, and a positive ANA. She has also responded to treatment with NSAIDs. The most likely diagnosis is oligoarticular JIA. This is the most common form of JIA and often responds well to treatment. The patient is followed up in Paediatric Rheumatology Clinic over the next year and she remains stable, with no further flare-ups of joint or eye symptoms.

Case history 11.2

An 18-year-old male is referred to the adult Rheumatology service. He has been under the Paediatric Rheumatology service for the previous 6 years since he was 12. He presented with weight loss, fevers, joint pains in his hips and knees and also a rash that coincided with his fever. He was diagnosed with systemic JIA and initially started on oral methotrexate. He developed severe nausea and vomiting with methotrexate, which was then switched to subcutaneous injections. Unfortunately, he was unable to tolerate injections as he continued to suffer from nausea and vomiting. The Rheumatology team spoke to him about how he was coping. He told the psychologist supporting the team that he was finding it difficult to cope with his diagnosis and schoolwork. He had aching and stiffness most mornings, especially in his hands and hips, which was lasting a few hours and was having to take a lot of time off school. The Consultant arranged X-rays of his hands and hips, which showed erosions in his wrists and both hips. She discussed changing his treatment for his JIA.

What would be the next best treatment option?

- Referral for bilateral hip replacements
- Counsel patient for TNF inhibitor biologic therapy
- Arrange steroid injection both hips
- Prescribe NSAIDs to control pain
- Refer to physiotherapy

The patient has been unable to tolerate methotrexate and has erosive disease on X-rays of his hands and hips, so has progressive JIA. He requires treatment escalation with TNF inhibitor therapy, which was started in the form of etanercept. Six months after starting this treatment, his symptoms were much improved and he was able to apply for a place at college. He was able to self-inject weekly after being taught how to do so, and remained in remission.

11.6 References

Colebatch-Bourn, A.N., Edwards, C.J., Collado, P. *et al.* (2015) EULAR-PReS points to consider for the use of imaging in the diagnosis and management of juvenile idiopathic arthritis in clinical practice. *Ann Rheum Dis.*, **74**: 1946–57.

Ravelli, A., Minoia, F., Davì, S. *et al.* (2016) 2016 Classification criteria for macrophage activation syndrome complicating systemic juvenile idiopathic arthritis: a European League Against Rheumatism/American College of Rheumatology/ Paediatric Rheumatology International Trials Organisation collaborative initiative. *Ann Rheum Dis.*, **68(3)**: 566–76.

Ringold, S., Weiss, P.F., Beukelman, T. *et al.* (2013) 2013 Update of the 2011 American College of Rheumatology recommendations for the treatment of juvenile idiopathic arthritis. *Arthritis Rheum.*, **65(10)**: 2499–2512.

Ringold, S., Angeles-Han, S.T., Beukelman, T. *et al.* (2019) 2019 American College of Rheumatology/Arthritis Foundation Guidelines for the treatment of juvenile idiopathic arthritis: therapeutic approaches for non-systemic polyarthritis, sacroiliitis, and enthesitis. *Arthritis Care Res.*, **71(6)**: 717–734.

NICE guidelines for biologic therapies in JIA

www.nice.org.uk/guidance/ta373

Appendix

Typical normal ranges for blood parameters

Full blood count

Hb:
- Male 120–180g/L
- Female 115–165g/L

WCC: $4–11 \times 10^9$/L

Platelets: $150–450 \times 10^9$/L

Neutrophils: $1.5–8.0 \times 10^9$/L

Lymphocytes: $1.1–4.0 \times 10^9$/L

Monocytes: $0.2–1.1 \times 10^9$/L

Eosinophils: $0.1–0.4 \times 10^9$/L

Basophils: $0–0.3 \times 10^9$/L

Inflammatory markers

ESR: 1–20mm/hour

CRP: 0–5mg/L

Renal function tests

Sodium: 133–146mmol/L

Potassium: 3.5–5.3mmol/L

Urea: 2.5–7.8mmol/L

Creatinine: 60–106μmol/L

eGFR: 89ml/min/1.73m^2

Multiply eGFR by 1.159 if patient is Afro-Caribbean. The eGFR calculation assumes a stable creatinine level. It is not valid if the creatinine levels are changing, or in certain patient groups, such as the malnourished, amputees and pregnant women. For further information see www.emrn.org.uk.

Liver function tests

Bilirubin: 0–21μmol/L

Alanine transaminase: 0–52U/L

Alkaline phosphatase: 30–160U/L

Albumin: 35–50g/L

Bone profile

Calcium: 2.2–2.6mmol/L

Phosphate: 0.8–1.5mmol/L

Adjusted calcium: 2.2–2.6mmol/L

25-hydroxyvitamin D: 50–174nmol/L

The National Osteoporosis Society Guidelines advise:

Serum 25(OH)D <25nmol/L is deficient

Serum 25(OH)D of 25–50nmol/L may be inadequate in some

Serum 25(OH)D >50nmol/L is sufficient for almost the whole population

Other biochemistry

Cholesterol: 3.3–5.2mmol/L

Ferritin: 30–400mcg/L

Folate: >20.0mcg/L

Triglyceride: 0.8–2.0mmol/L

Thyroid-stimulating hormone (TSH): 0.27–4.20mU/L

Vitamin B12: 180–999ng/L

Uric acid: 200–430μmol/L

Immunology

Complement C3: 0.75–1.65g/L

Complement C4: 0.14–0.54g/L

Anti-CCP antibodies: 0–7U/ml

RhF: 0–20 IU/ml

ANAs with a significant titre of between 1:160 and 1:2560 is considered to indicate a significant result. A more detailed analysis of ANAs includes the dsDNA antibody titre. In typical cases of lupus, a value of >200U/ml is considered to be elevated. Levels of dsDNA can be used to correlate with clinical disease activity and response to treatment.

Different laboratories also have their own reference ranges for autoantibodies to the following antibody assays, which are associated with specific autoimmune conditions.

Anti-Ro and -La antibodies: Sjögren's syndrome

ANA, dsDNA: SLE

RNP: SLE (cerebral involvement), systemic sclerosis, polymyositis, mixed connective tissue disease

Anti-Sm antibodies: SLE renal involvement, mixed connective tissue disease

Anti-centromere antibodies: limited systemic sclerosis

Anti-Scl 70 antibodies (targeted to topoisomerase 1): diffuse systemic sclerosis

Anti-synthetase antibodies: include anti Jo-1, PL-7 and PL-12, associated with myositis

Index